The Power and Limitation of Kriya Yoga

Prof. A.N. Pandey

ISBN: 1537567403
ISBN-13: 978-1537567402

DEDICATION

This book is dedicated to the scientists and spiritual masters of the world in order to explore the hidden potential power in them for discovery of new concepts to be used by mankind. This book is the alternative source of erasing diseases and maintaining the vibrant aspects of mind.

CONTENTS

ACKNOWLEDGMENTS

I (Author) acknowledge the valuable contribution of Swami Satyadharama of Bihar school of Yoga. He has very effectively discovered the theme of Veda and kept the same in a book form known as Yoga Chudamani Upanishad (Crown Jewel of Yoga). I offer my Pranam to him for such a valuable job. His work will certainly guide the seekers in the field of Yoga and Spirituality.

I bow my head on the lotus feet of Paramhansa Yogananda Ji for his discovery of Kriya Yoga in the easy form. Many seekers would have got benefitted by his blessings. This book is intended to remind the practitioner of Kriya yoga for obtaining the benefits if followed correctly. This is because; most of the practitioners do not remember the basic theme of Kriya yoga.

I also offer my Pranam to Dr. H.R. Nagendra, Chancellor of SVYASA (World Class Yoga University at Bengaluru) for his guidance in the field of Yogic concept. This book is outcome of the joint efforts carried in the field of Kriya yoga and research work at Spiritual Awareness Program (SAP), Hyderabad.

1. INTRODUCTION

Kriya Yoga, widely known in Eastern Part of India, is given in different forms to aspirants by different Gurus. In Guru Shishya Parampra (tradition of Master – disciple), is existing in established traditions and the same is being transferred from one Guru to another. For example, Kriya Yoga was transmitted from Baba Ji to Lahari Mahashya to Yukteswar Swami to Paramhansa Yogananda Ji.

But another form of Kriya Yoga is also developed by different Acharya based on their experiences. For example, Kriya Yoga given by SKY (Simplified Kundalini Yoga) in the form of "Kaya Kalpa" (to retain the youth hood of the body) and other associates of Yogada Satsang differ in certain extent.

This made me conscious to know the actual or original concepts of Kriya Yoga described in Veda or in Upanishad. Fortunately, "Yoga Chudamani Upanishad" also known as Crown Jewels of Yoga" provides the clear concepts of Kriya Yoga related to its basic principles, purpose, methodology, benefits, Limitation with precaution.

1.1 What is Yoga Chudamani Upanishad?

Upanishads related to Yoga existed many years before Yoga Chudamani Upanishad came into existence. Yogic Upanishads deal with major aspects like Kundalini, Laya, Nada, Mantra and Hatha. The Yogic Upanishads were composed after "Yoga Sutra" of Patanjali and form an important part of Yogic literature. The earliest Yogic Upanishads are certainly Pre-Patanjali & are composed between the completion of Vedic hymns around 1000BC and classical Yoga period which arose 300BC. In the early Upanishad like Brihadaranyaka and Chandogya, different Vidyas or meditative disciplines are described, but nowhere were they codified as in Patanjali Yoga sutra.

Yoga Chudamani is crown jewels of Yoga. It is comprised of 121 mantras which deal with the practices of Kundalini Yoga as a means to attain the heights of Vedanta philosophy. The author and origins of Yoga Chudamani text probably emerge from "Sama – Veda", probably dates back to the period between 700 - 1000AD. Some scholars have related the practical content of their text with Hatha Yoga.

Yoga Chudamani is a manual of Higher Sadhana which is meant for advanced and initiated aspirants. While describing the mantra, the text points out the necessary means of transformation which leads to an experience of the deeper aspects of Yoga sadhana and it culminates in the experience of consciousness and self realization. This way, the text becomes a practical and experiential proof of the compatibility of Yoga and Vedanta.

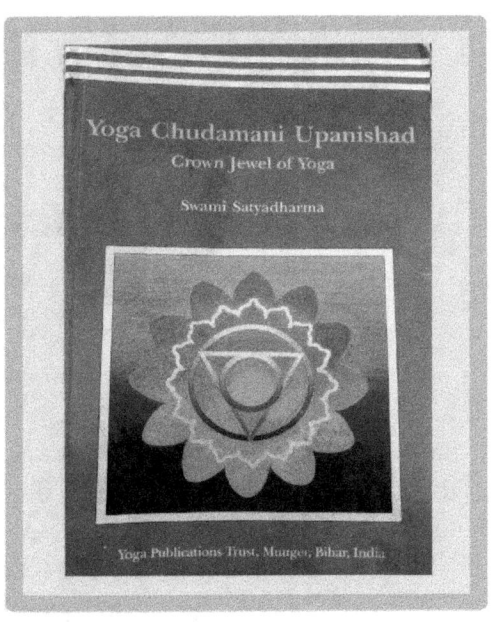

Veda is original text to describe all prevailing knowledge including yogic knowledge in general and Kriya Yoga in particular. Upanishad (the brief of Veda) provides all basic principles and knowledge of Kriya Yoga by describing different combination of Astang Yoga like Asana, Pranayama, bandha and Mudra. All four aspects have to be synchronized in order to get full benefits of Kriya Yoga. In absence of one or two, Kriya Yoga will provide harmful effect emplace of its benefits.

2. WHY AUTHOR GOT INVOLVED?

Author is practicing Kriya Yoga related to Special Bhramari technique, Simplified Kundalini Yoga (SKY) dealing with "Kaya Kalpa" and Kriya Yoga of Yogada Satsang. Diving in the depth of Kriya Yoga described in Yoga Chudamani Upanishad, Author found an alarming mantra in the text. There is a warning in one of the Mantra (MN-70) of Yoga Chudamani Upanishad that Maha Mudra (the main technique of Kriya Yoga) is very powerful and it should not be given to anyone. This mantra led Author to know the depth of Kriya Yoga processes further; where mistakes are likely to happen during performance and what will be the consequences (results) after mistakes? Because of the caution (warning), Kriya Yoga is not supposed to be given just like that to everyone without knowing the eligibility of the aspirants.

In the age of internet, nothing can be kept secret;

hence it is better to know its boons and banes fully while practicing the same (Kriya Yoga). Last few years, Kriya Yoga has become the hot cake in spiritual world as the aspirants have been given the exposure of its benefits only. The banes of Kriya Yoga (if not practiced correctly) have not been elaborated; hence the performer of Kriya yoga might get in trouble in due course. However, Yogada satsang provides all precautionary measures if the same (Kriya Yoga) is given by authentic masters. Because of curiosity and urgency to take up Kriya Yoga by the aspirants, there is probability to do some mistakes while practicing the same; even though, correct methodology has been given by the master.

This book is an eye opener to all the Sadhakas of Kriya Yoga. This provides the inbuilt corrective approach in the minds of Sadhaka, whether the method adopted in Kriya Yoga is fully correct or any mistakes is being carried out? This book also brings mile stone or yard stick to the seeker by cropping its results in terms of benefits. This book works like an alarming bell against its caution or warning provided in MN -70 of Yoga Chudamani Upanishad. To gain the maximum benefits of Kriya Yoga, the book is placed before the reader without having any like and Dislikes against any cult or master of Kriya Yoga.

■

3. BINDU (NUCLEI) IN THE CONTEXT OF MODERN SCIENCE

The nuclei (Bindu) are the nodal points of energy (Shakti, Prakriti, and Prana), space (Shiva, Purusha, and Mind) and consciousness (Brahma, soul or Jiva). Hence this consists of consciousness defined in science, yoga and Vedanta. This immerges from the transcendental state to the cellular level of human being by bringing all possible aspects of cosmic intelligence from supreme reality to cells level of human being. In three bodies level (causal, subtle and gross body level) it passes the information by coordinating the existing energy and space at different centers.

The coordination of consciousness (Bindu) along with energy and space have been defined by science in classical theory (classical mechanics) and termed as i) High Order theory ii) Biological theory and iii) Global work place theory. The classical theory is based on the consciousness defined in quantum mechanics. This means classical theory corresponds to artificial intelligence where as quantum theory corresponds to cosmic intelligence.

Similar concepts have already experienced by the Indian seers who have reached the depth of Yoga and Vedanta. As per yogic concepts four dimensions of consciousness have been defined and they are Vishwa, Rajas, Pragnya and Serva Sakshi corresponding to the Vedantic concepts of consciousness. In Vedanta, the consciousness has been defined as individual, cosmic, absolute and indwelling consciousness.

The term Bindu (nuclei) clarifies that the holistic approach at any level depends on three characteristics like energy, space and consciousness. This means the integration of energy, space and consciousness (all together) can be termed as Bindu.

3.1 Creation (Birth of an Individual)

Upanishad describes that creation (birth) of an individual happens because of a nucleus (Bindu) immerges from supreme reality and the same immerges as an existence. The diagram explains that Parabindu (shown as no.1) creates Shiva (space) and Shakti (energy) to initiate the creation in pure Spiritual (Adhyatmik) dimension. Further the Nucleus (Bindu) passes through subtle (Daivik) dimension where the causal body returns to take rebirth depending upon stored imprints (Sanchit karma) and imprints to be erased by enjoyment or suffering (Prarabdha karma).

In gross (Bhoutik) dimension the nucleus comes to Hiranyagarba consisting soul, five elements as an energy and inner instrument (Antahkarna). In biological term, Nucleus means 'a structure present in most cells, containing the genetic material along with the original Bindu (combination of consciousness, energy and space)'. This nucleus (Bindu) further becomes the two nuclei (Bindu) at the time of growing causal body, subtle body and gross body in mother's womb. After the birth again the Jiva (Individual soul) experiencing the growth of causal body, subtle body and physical (gross) body till the youth hood is achieved. The image briefly describes the formation of nuclei during creation and return of the same (nuclei) during dissolution.

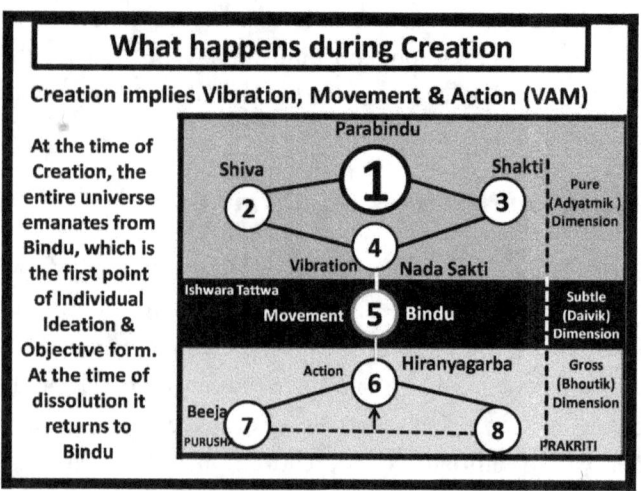

For clarity of the reader, it must be noted that rajas and Bindu are the two forms of original Bindu (Nuclei) during inception in mother's womb. While developing from causal to subtle and further Physical body in mother's womb and also the development before youth hood, the original nucleus become two (Bindu and Rajas). Bindu stays at Bindu Visarga (the top back of the head) and Rajas stays at Swadisthana when youth hood is completed. Bindu is also known as consciousness, Purusha, Shiva, Moon, Mind and Ida. Likewise, Rajas is termed as Energy, Prakriti, Shakti, Sun, Prana and Pingla. These terms are used while evolving at different body in Spiritual Journey.

3.2 How Nuclei work on cells of human beings?

Bindu (Nuclei) consisting all points (cosmic intelligence) of creation emerging from almighty. It transfers the energy and space characteristics of supreme reality to cells of human beings for keeping healthy body and mind. While passing the growth from causal to subtle body and finally to the gross body, the cells become the coordinating agency between existing vital force and energy from the soul or supreme reality.

The image explains that every cell of Body depends on the nerves and blood vessels for substance & integration with the rest of the body. This clarifies that whatever substance comes in the cell will get integrated throughout the body. For example, cells get the information of cosmic intelligence and will integrate the same in artificial intelligence provided the purity of the mind is fully obtained. This means that Bindu is not only the seed but also the vital source of life cellular level which sustains and links every cell of the body.

At cell level, the Bindu brings the transcendental

concept of creation down to the physical plane for Jagrat, Swapna & Sushupti states experience and also their corresponding mental states and perception. In three physical states (awakened, dream and deep sleep) the corresponding experiences are linked with the three mental states (conscious, subconscious and unconscious states of mind). Bindu as consciousness brings the transcendental concepts (unknown concepts of supreme reality) in three physical states of human being as intuition depending on the purity of each level of mind.

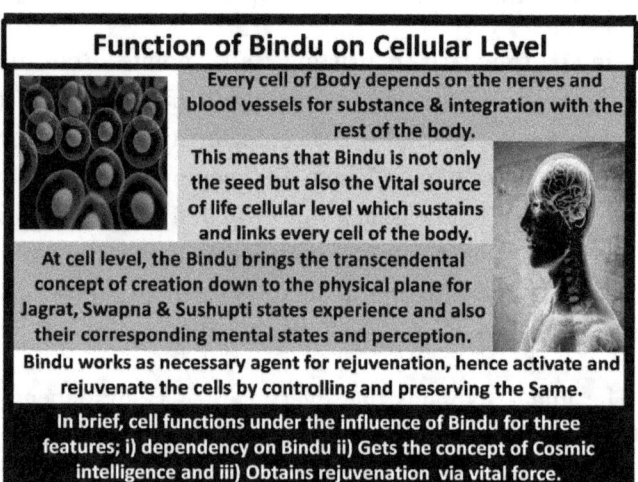

Bindu works as necessary agent for rejuvenation hence activate and rejuvenate the cells by controlling and preserving the same. This clarifies that Bindu (Nuclei) is an agent for each physical and mental state of individual for coordinating the vital force and concerned conscious state of mind together. In brief, cell functions under the influence of Bindu for three features i) dependency on Bindu (Nuclei) ii) Gets the concept of

Cosmic Intelligence and iii) Obtains rejuvenation via vital force.

3.3 Nucleus gets divided to form level of two minds

The main nucleus (Bindu) gets divided into two Bindu existing at top back of the head and another at Swadisthana Chakra in the process of reaching youth hood. The stability of the nuclei (Bindu) happens while formation of Causal, Subtle and Gross body. Position of energy centers at different chakra is briefly explained in the image. The Rajas (lower level of mind) will exist either at Swadisthana or Manipura Chakra; but both are not the conducive position of lower mind for the growth.

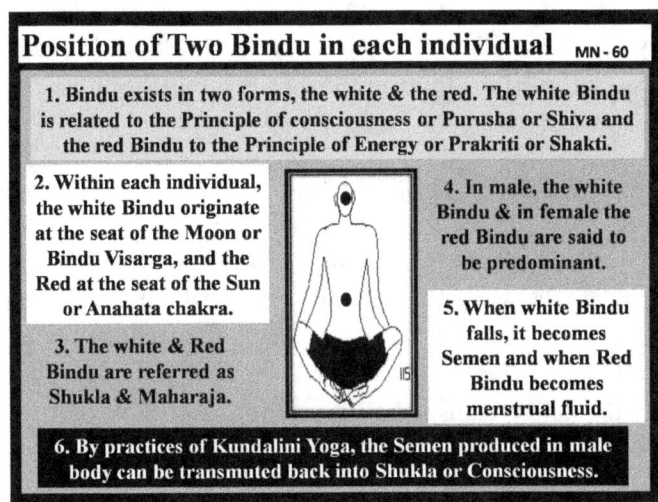

Position of Two Bindu in each individual   MN - 60

1. Bindu exists in two forms, the white & the red. The white Bindu is related to the Principle of consciousness or Purusha or Shiva and the red Bindu to the Principle of Energy or Prakriti or Shakti.

2. Within each individual, the white Bindu originate at the seat of the Moon or Bindu Visarga, and the Red at the seat of the Sun or Anahata chakra.

3. The white & Red Bindu are referred as Shukla & Maharaja.

4. In male, the white Bindu & in female the red Bindu are said to be predominant.

5. When white Bindu falls, it becomes Semen and when Red Bindu becomes menstrual fluid.

6. By practices of Kundalini Yoga, the Semen produced in male body can be transmuted back into Shukla or Consciousness.

In human beings, Bindu exists in two forms, the white & the red. The white Bindu is related to the Principle of consciousness or Purusha or Shiva and the red Bindu to the Principle of Energy or Prakriti or Shakti. In scientific term, White Bindu is known as a space and Red Bindu is known as energy.

Within each individual, the white Bindu originate at the seat of the Moon or Bindu Visarga (top back of the head), and the Red at the seat of the Sun or Anahata chakra. Manipura chakra is responsible for burning the nectar (Amrit) dropping in each individual. That is why the existence of red Bindu at Manipura is not advisable. The white & Red Bindu are referred as Shukla & Maharaja in Vedic scripture. But the same can be referred as space and energy in scientific terminology. In male, the white Bindu & in female the red Bindu are said to be predominant. When white Bindu falls, it becomes Semen and when Red Bindu becomes menstrual fluid. By practices of Kriya Yoga, the Semen produced in male body can be transmuted back into Shukla or Consciousness.

3.3.1 The division of Bindu

The image describes that the Original Bindu is divided into two types, Pandara (white) and Lohita (red). The white is called Shukla and the red is called Maharaja. This is described in MN-60 of Yoga Chudamani Upanishad. The mantra indicates that the main nucleus (Bindu) originates from nature (Prakriti) who is the manager of creation. This nucleus is supposed to have complete essential aspects or ingredients (like soul, elements and inner instrument) of life journey. The Bindu gets divided because of Sanchit and Prarabdha karma and effect of Genes from Parents.

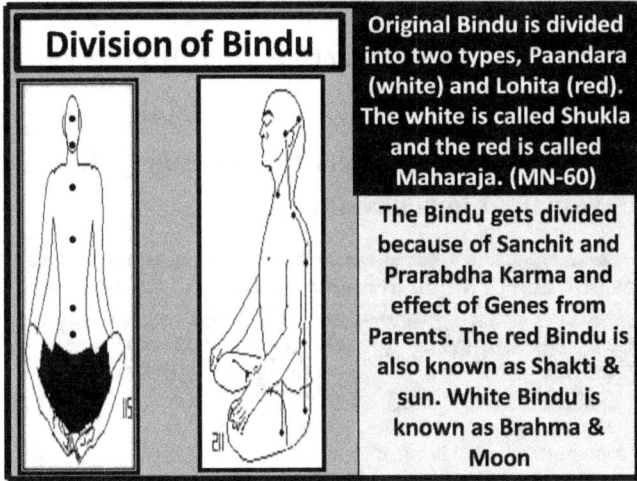

Division of Bindu

Original Bindu is divided into two types, Paandara (white) and Lohita (red). The white is called Shukla and the red is called Maharaja. (MN-60)

The Bindu gets divided because of Sanchit and Prarabdha Karma and effect of Genes from Parents. The red Bindu is also known as Shakti & sun. White Bindu is known as Brahma & Moon

The red Bindu is also known as Shakti & sun. White Bindu is known as Brahman & Moon. In scientific term the White Bindu is responsible for the functional aspects of space (having least possible energy). The strength of White Bindu can be measured by the purity of Chitta (one of the aspects of internal instrument). The Red Bindu signifies the energy (having least possible space) and can be measured with the help of its (energy) purity.

3.4 Need for correction

In absence of detailed knowledge of Maha Mudra will not unveil the importance and benefit of Kriya yoga. This is because, there is basic difference of energy (the higher and lower mental energy) distribution in men and women. This is also true because of masculine and feminine characteristics of these two genders having different chromosome. The men and women naturally, will have different characteristics of energy (prana) governing system. The point has been clarified by analyzing the existence of nuclei (Bindu) for men and women.

3.4.1 Different characteristics of energy in men and women at lower chakra

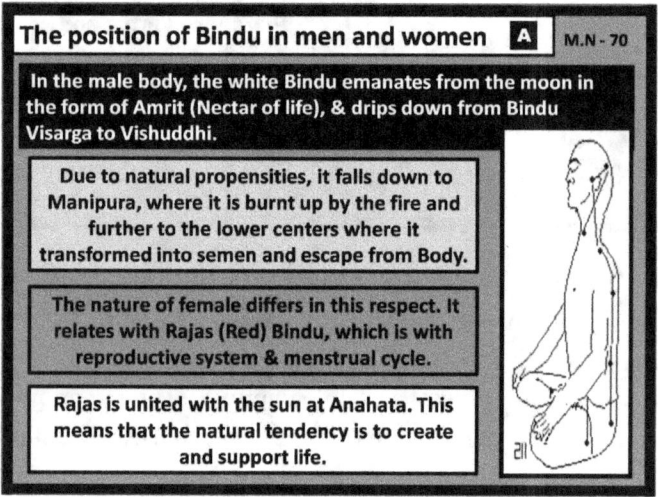

The position of Bindu in men and women

In the male body, the white Bindu emanates from the moon in the form of Amrit (Nectar of life), & drips down from Bindu Visarga to Vishuddhi.

Due to natural propensities, it falls down to Manipura, where it is burnt up by the fire and further to the lower centers where it transformed into semen and escape from Body.

The nature of female differs in this respect. It relates with Rajas (Red) Bindu, which is with reproductive system & menstrual cycle.

Rajas is united with the sun at Anahata. This means that the natural tendency is to create and support life.

In the male body, the white Bindu emanates from the moon in the form of Amrit (Nectar of life), & drips down from Bindu Visarga to Manipura or Vishuddhi. Due to natural propensities, it falls down to Manipura, where it is burnt up by the fire and further to the lower centers where it transformed into semen and escape from Body. The nature of female differs in this respect. It relates with Rajas (Red) Bindu, which is with reproductive system & menstrual cycle. Rajas is united with the sun at Anahata this means that the natural tendency is to create and support life.

Without raising the Bindu up to Anahata, a man can live normal life as energy requirement by the senses is met with the help of food, vitamins, minerals and the required amount of rest. The replacement of functional energy is also equipped by deep sleep. However, if men are able to uplift the lower Bindu (Rajas) up to Anahata chakra and retain the Bindu at that chakra, he will be able to have the better personality.

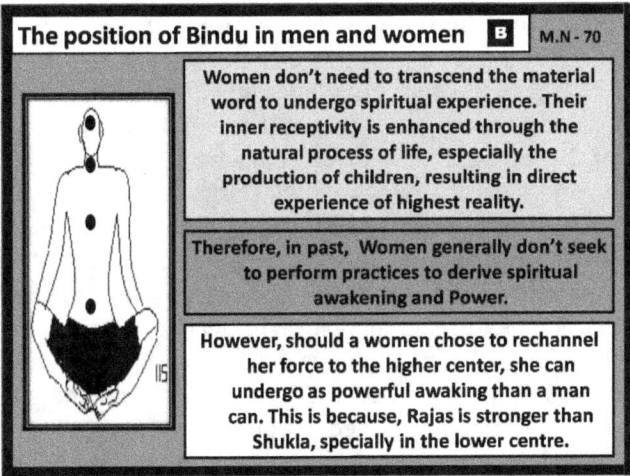

The position of Bindu in men and women **B** M.N - 70

Women don't need to transcend the material word to undergo spiritual experience. Their inner receptivity is enhanced through the natural process of life, especially the production of children, resulting in direct experience of highest reality.

Therefore, in past, Women generally don't seek to perform practices to derive spiritual awakening and Power.

However, should a women chose to rechannel her force to the higher center, she can undergo as powerful awaking than a man can. This is because, Rajas is stronger than Shukla, specially in the lower centre.

Women don't need to transcend the material word to undergo spiritual experience. Their inner receptivity is enhanced through the natural process of life, especially the production of children, resulting in direct experience of highest reality. Therefore, in past, Women generally don't seek to perform practices to derive spiritual awakening and Power.

However, should women choose to rechanneling her force to the higher center, she can undergo as powerful awaking than a man can. This is because, Rajas is stronger than Shukla, especially in the lower centre. This indicates that the women can reach at higher chakra easily and can also be able to retain the nucleus (Bindu) effectively compared to a man. For example, a man has to struggle more to raise White Bindu at lower centers and also to reach at the original center at Bindu Visarga (top back of the head) compared to a women.

3.5 Why to take the corrective measures?

To take the corrective measures for enhancing the Rajas Bindu in men and women, there are many methods to uplift and hold the lower mind or Bindu at upper chakra and also finally at Bindu Visarga (top back of the head). In yogic practice Bahirang yoga provides the methodology to reach the top back of the head. It is interesting to note that if lower nucleus stays at or below Manipura chakra, the people will lead a normal life under the grip of certain physical ailments. If the nucleus (Bindu) of lower mind or energy exists at Anahata and above & the same is retained at higher chakra, the people will have better personality in their performances. If the people are able to retain the lower Bindu above Vishuddhi chakra, they will be in a position to have the vibrant life. Finally if the lower Bindu (Rajas) is merged with Shukla (White Bindu) at Bindu Visarga, the people will be Divine and will be in a position to take the quantum jump in the domain of supreme reality or transcendental body.

4. PURPOSE OF KRIYA YOGA

There are three ways to uplift our consciousness (the nucleus resulting because of two forces). One method could be balancing the two forces (force related to prana and mind flowing in Pingla and Ida path respectively) and get the nuclei (resultant) uplifted at higher center. Second method could be worked upon either of the two forces (which are inter linked) and then to obtain the nucleus (consciousness) uplifted. These two methods can be practiced with the help of Asana, Pranayama and Pratyahara steps of Astang Yoga.

The third method is little different than the above two. In this method the Bindu (Nuclei) as a consciousness which normally take the path of Sushumna. If the nucleus, is moved by any means in upward direction and kept controlled there for longer time; that kind of method defines the purpose of Kriya yoga. That is why, Kriya yoga is taken as a different subject compared to normal Astang yoga; though, the steps (like Asana, Pranayama, Bandha and Mudra) followed in Kriya yoga are the part of Astang yoga.

4.1 Why Kriya Yoga is taken as corrective measures for progressive life?

Kriya yoga is a corrective tool to achieve dynamic life in general and spiritual life in particular for evolution. Atheist and Theist do believe that there is a great role of nature (Prakriti) to create individual's life or existence. While creation, all essential aspects of life comes in a Nuclei (Bindu) form, Nuclei (Bindu) consists of higher mind (space) and also lower mind (energy). The higher mind is full of Antahkarna with least possible energy stays at top back of the head; whereas lower mind consists of maximum energy and stays randomly at lower chakra (mostly at Swadisthana chakra) for common man. The Kriya yoga is a methodology to raise the lower mind (energy) from lower chakra to higher chakra (distributor of energy for the specific region) so as to achieve the dynamic personality and also to achieve the divinity for the individual.

The diagram shows energy level at different chakras. This is bound to happen in day to day life depending on individual's nature, family and social atmosphere, financial condition and educational level.

Actual source of Bindu is the higher centers of the Brain, in the region of Bindu Visarga (top back of the head). Due to influence of Desire and Passion, the Bindu falls down the lower region. The falling depends on the intensity of desire and passions. For example, in the young age desire and passions are very high. That is why the nuclei (Bindu) during youth hood stay at lower centers.

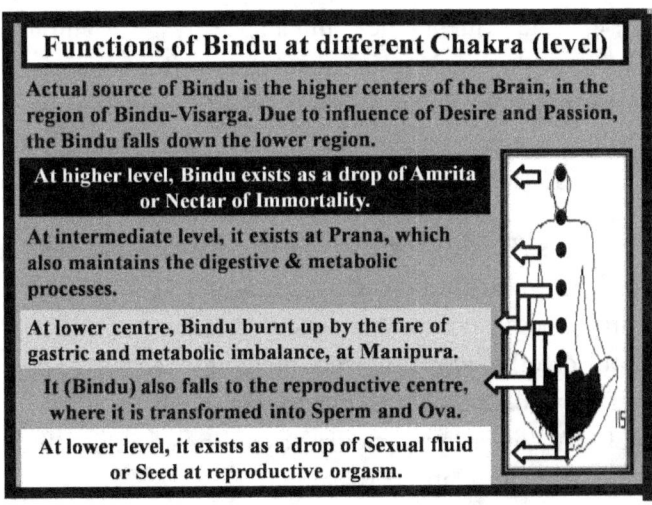

Functions of Bindu at different Chakra (level)

Actual source of Bindu is the higher centers of the Brain, in the region of Bindu-Visarga. Due to influence of Desire and Passion, the Bindu falls down the lower region.

At higher level, Bindu exists as a drop of Amrita or Nectar of Immortality.

At intermediate level, it exists at Prana, which also maintains the digestive & metabolic processes.

At lower centre, Bindu burnt up by the fire of gastric and metabolic imbalance, at Manipura.

It (Bindu) also falls to the reproductive centre, where it is transformed into Sperm and Ova.

At lower level, it exists as a drop of Sexual fluid or Seed at reproductive orgasm.

At higher level, Bindu exists as a drop of Amrita or Nectar of Immortality. This happens whenever the Bindu (the controller) of lower mind gets merged with the Bindu of higher mind at Bindu Visarga. As long as union of two Bindu (lower and higher) exists, there will be the formation of Amrit (Nectar).

At intermediate level, it exists at Anahata chakra as Prana and further maintains the digestive & metabolic processes. The Anahata center is the source of main Prana. At the center, the prana (inherent vital force) comes along with air and gets distributed in two parts. The upper part of the Prana works for Vishuddhi chakra and also for central nervous system. The lower part of

Prana passes through digestive system (like Samana Prana) and moves lower region of the body like Apana Prana.

At lower centre, Bindu gets burnt up by the fire of gastric and metabolic imbalance, at Manipura. However, the center is also responsible for good digestion when Samana prana is sufficient. This is possible when Apana prana is weak or having Urdhvagati (upward direction) to assist Samana prana.

Nucleus (Bindu) also falls to the reproductive centre, where it is transformed into Sperm and Ova. This is a natural process and to overcome this, Kriya yoga is very helpful or effective. If correct method of Kriya yoga is not followed, there is likelihood of harm in place of benefit. At lower level, it exists as a drop of Sexual fluid or Seed at reproductive orgasm.

4.2 Benefits of Kriya yoga

The practice of Kriya yoga provides many benefits like retention of healthy cells, reduction of ageing, keeping proper digestive system and elimination of diseases. In brief the image describes the main features of the benefit.

Retention of Bindu is prescribed for three reasons to have its benefits. i) Bindu is the source of creation and of individual manifestation & maintenance of life. This means, the retention of Bindu leads to Immortal life but the loss leads to degeneration of cells (body) & death. This is because, when retention of Bindu at higher points or chakra is not maintained, then the cells are not getting rejuvenated and more cells die compared to new number of cells generating in the body.

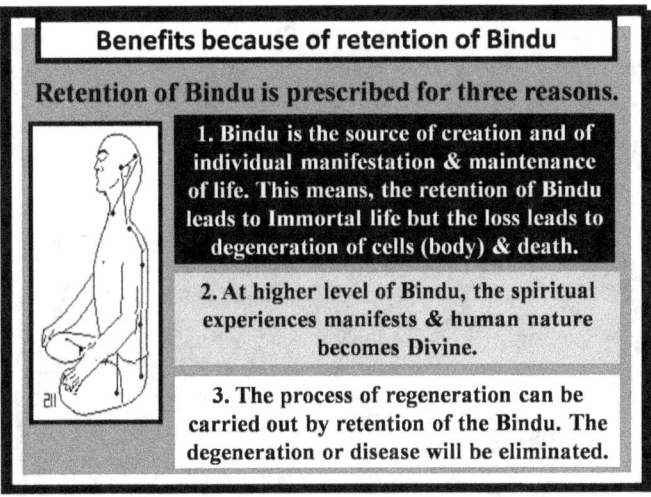

Benefits because of retention of Bindu

Retention of Bindu is prescribed for three reasons.

1. Bindu is the source of creation and of individual manifestation & maintenance of life. This means, the retention of Bindu leads to Immortal life but the loss leads to degeneration of cells (body) & death.

2. At higher level of Bindu, the spiritual experiences manifests & human nature becomes Divine.

3. The process of regeneration can be carried out by retention of the Bindu. The degeneration or disease will be eliminated.

ii) At higher level of Bindu, the spiritual experiences manifests & human nature becomes Divine. At that point, the divinity is experienced when lower Bindu (Rajas or sun or prana) is merged with white Bindu (mind, moon, and shiva) at Bindu Visarga. iii) The process of regeneration can be carried out by retention of the Bindu. The degeneration or disease will be eliminated. This is the main principle of Kriya yoga. This indicates that at any stage or any age of human life, the Kriya yoga can be practiced perfectly to raise the lower Bindu at higher chakra and also to unite the Rajas (lower Bindu) with Shukla (higher Bindu) at Bindu Visarga.

4.3 Proper stability of nuclei makes dynamic personality

It is interesting to note that the preservation of Bindu at different chakra yields different skills and special characteristics of the personality. This is because; the vital fluid (which normally remains at two lower chakras) works as energy drainer. When vital force along with Apana prana is raised and retained at higher chakra, the inner potentiality of the individual blossom up.

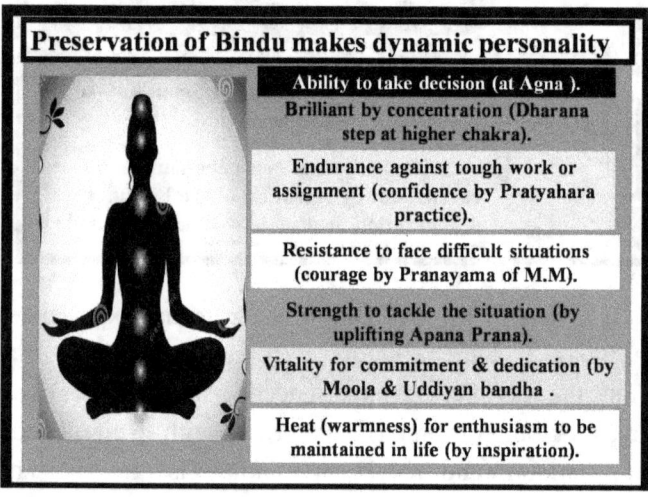

Preservation of Bindu makes dynamic personality

Ability to take decision (at Agna).

Brilliant by concentration (Dharana step at higher chakra).

Endurance against tough work or assignment (confidence by Pratyahara practice).

Resistance to face difficult situations (courage by Pranayama of M.M).

Strength to tackle the situation (by uplifting Apana Prana).

Vitality for commitment & dedication (by Moola & Uddiyan bandha .

Heat (warmness) for enthusiasm to be maintained in life (by inspiration).

For example, the individual develops the Ability to take decision when Bindu is raised and retained at Agna chakra. At this point, the lower mental state (represented by Rajas) becomes fully balanced and the consciousness at this moment becomes capable to move in the psychic channel.

The practitioner of Kriya Yoga (Maha Mudra)

becomes brilliant as they can focus on the single subject at a time by developing the art of concentration. This is also achieved whenever the lower mind is raised up to frontal portion of the brain. This is achieved by adopting the principle of Dharana (concentration) of Astang yoga.

The practitioner of Maha Mudra and Yoni Mudra becomes internally tough to face the time consuming works in day to day life. This can be ensured when the follower of Kriya yoga achieved endurance against tough work or assignment by practicing the technique of withdrawal (Pratyahara) indicated in Kriya yoga. It is interesting to note that withdrawal practice of Astang yoga helps the user to become more confident. This is the theme of the management course and the students of MBA are trained to be more confident in day to day work while dealing with the associates.

Another achievement for being dynamic is to become courageous. Kriya yoga builds sufficient strength in the individual to become resistant for facing the difficult situations. This can be achieved from the Pranayama steps given in Kriya yoga (Maha Mudra and Yoni Mudra) practice.

The procedure of Asana and Pranayama described in Maha Mudra and Yoni Mudra is very important and the same should be followed carefully by providing sufficient time for practice. This in turn, uplifts the Apana prana (lower energy) to activate Jathragni (the fire of digestive organs) and yields sufficient strength for Worldly and Spiritual works. This is also important for providing the good appetite in individual.

The practice of Moola bandha and Uddiyan bandha while performing Maha mudra should be done correctly so as to raise the vital force to achieve the sense of commitment and dedication for day to day work. The practice of these two bandha also helps to overcome procrastination; which is an essential factor for modern work place management. Kriya yoga helps to achieve the essential strength of prana (energy) so that Sadhaka feels warm enough to maintain the enthusiastic aspects of inspiration while interacting at family, at field of work, with friends and relatives and also while developing the self.

4.4 How to achieve the vibrant life?

To achieve all round benefits in physical, mental and spiritual domain, the better regular and disciplined life style are the main criteria. Generally, disciplined life style is followed by top scientists, thinkers, writers, poets, musicians and dancers. Regular and disciplined life style will certainly enhance the lower level of mind (the nucleus of Rajas or Shakti or Sun etc) at higher Chakra but the same will not provide the essential and utmost benefits of artificial intelligence. The artificial intelligence can be defined by three dimensions of consciousness like individual, cosmic and absolute consciousness. The dynamic personality in the respective field can achieve any of the three consciousnesses but are likely to descend down.

Yogic practice of Special Pranayama like Chandra Bheda and Surya Bheda Pranayama are very helpful to raise the lower nucleus (lower mind) to upper centers depending on the perfection. Similarly, Moola, Uddiyan, Jalandhar Bandha will help to transform and control the stability of lower nucleus of Mind (energy) at higher level. Next very effective processes to merge the lower nucleus (Bindu) with upper Nucleus (higher mind) are Maha Mudra and Yoni mudra. These two Mudras can be performed easily by discipline Sadhaka and they are the parts of main Kriya Yoga.

However, Khechari Mudra is the best possible way of Kriya Yoga but it is very difficult to practice. Some of the cults of Kriya Yoga provide the emphasis on Khechari Mudra. The image describes the utility of Khechari Mudra for stopping the fall of Bindu (nuclei), but the same is very difficult to be performed.

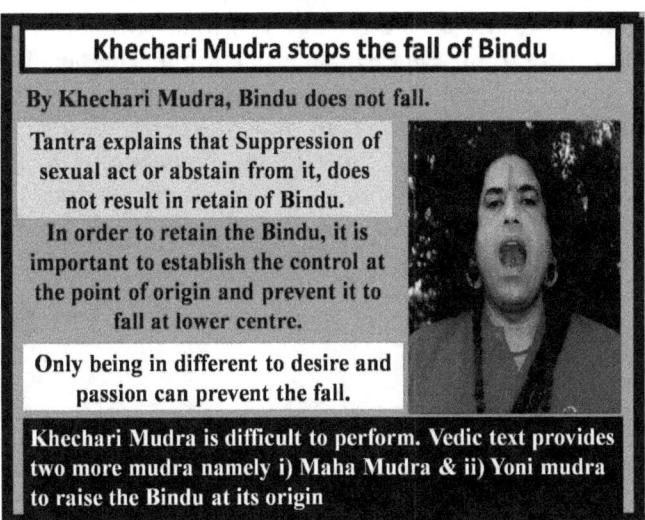

Khechari Mudra stops the fall of Bindu

By Khechari Mudra, Bindu does not fall.

Tantra explains that Suppression of sexual act or abstain from it, does not result in retain of Bindu.

In order to retain the Bindu, it is important to establish the control at the point of origin and prevent it to fall at lower centre.

Only being in different to desire and passion can prevent the fall.

Khechari Mudra is difficult to perform. Vedic text provides two more mudra namely i) Maha Mudra & ii) Yoni mudra to raise the Bindu at its origin

Tantra explains that Suppression of sexual act or abstain from it, does not result in retain of Bindu. Yoga and tantra explains not to have restraints forcibly but to achieve the aim (from Kam to Ram) should be practiced with the help of Asana, Pranayama, Bandha and Mudra.

In order to retain the Bindu, it is important to establish the control at the point of origin and prevent it to fall at lower centre. Khechari Mudra holds the original Bindu at Bindu Visarga. Only being in different to desire and passion can prevent the fall. This is because, desire makes the stability of higher mind weak and passion the lower mind further weak. This means that stability of higher mind (Bindu) and lower mind (Rajas Bindu) becomes weak because of desire and passion respectively.

Khechari Mudra is difficult to perform. Vedic text provides two more mudra namely i) Maha Mudra & ii) Yoni mudra to raise the Bindu at its origin. The benefits of Khechari Mudra can also be obtained with the help of Maha Mudra and Yoni mudra (being easier to practice). That is why, most of the branches of Kriya yoga advocate the practice of these two Mudras by combining Asana, Pranayama, Bandha and mudra (Maha Bheda mudra) together.

5. PRINCIPLE OF KRIYA YOGA

The main principle of Kriya yoga is to lift and merge the Red Bindu (signifies the lower mind) with White Bindu (signifies the higher mind) so as to become divine. This means that being divine is the platform for interaction of transcendental body (higher body) which is also known as indwelling consciousness (Sakshi Chaitanya). In brief the purpose of Kriya yoga can be summarized in two steps like i) to lift or raise the Red Bindu at higher chakra and ii) to merge both the Bindu at Bindu Visarga (top back of the head).

Kriya Yoga is given in two phases. First Maha Mudra technique is introduced and secondly Yoni Mudra or Shanmukhi Mudra is given. These two main steps are followed in Yogada Satsang. In the case of Special Bhramari and Kaya Kalpa techniques, similar kind of methodology is followed as adopted in Yogada Satsang. The process adopted in Kriya yoga (as described in MN-65 of Maha Mudra) provides the emphasis that combination of four like Asana, Pranayama, bandha and Mudra of Astang Yoga are must to crop the benefits. Ignoring or leaving one of the steps will not provide the desired result. This is because; these steps are also adopted to raise the nuclei of lower mental energy at higher level.

5.1 The first principle of Kriya yoga is to uplift the lower mind

The stability of red and white Bindu, at Anahata chakra and top back of the head, can provide sound physical and mental health. However, this will not make the people to develop their own personality for Worldly affairs and also to understand the unknown dimensions of spirituality. This is because, red Bindu consists of female characteristics of mind and male Bindu represents the masculine characteristics of the mind. Unless, both are developed and made equal in characteristics at particular point, the personality will not be stable. This also signifies the concept of Ardha Narishwar (half male and half female characteristics) to obtain sustainable (Purnta) dimension of a creation.

To explain the position of Nuclei in normal person, the analysis has been carried out and the same is summarized in the diagram. The image explains the effect of Bindu at different chakra to achieve different dimensions of personality.

At Vishuddhi chakra the Bindu is of Sattvik nature, nectarine & illumine in characteristics. This means the people possessing Bindu at this chakra will have vibrant personality. At Manipura chakra Bindu gets burnt up as it falls because of desires & passion and also having Rajas nature. To avoid or eliminate the fall, Rat race should be avoided. This can also be prevented by uplifting Apana prana and merging the same with Samana prana. At Manipura, the fire element represents Rajas (The dynamic quality of life); which can be modified by adopting the path of simple living and high thinking.

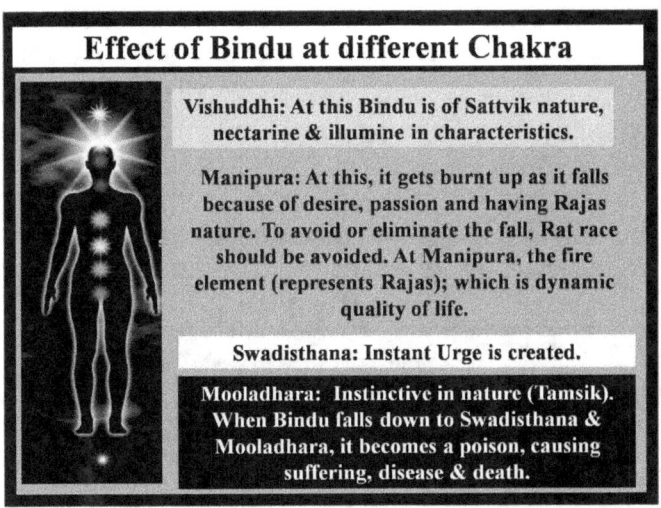

Effect of Bindu at different Chakra

Vishuddhi: At this Bindu is of Sattvik nature, nectarine & illumine in characteristics.

Manipura: At this, it gets burnt up as it falls because of desire, passion and having Rajas nature. To avoid or eliminate the fall, Rat race should be avoided. At Manipura, the fire element (represents Rajas); which is dynamic quality of life.

Swadisthana: Instant Urge is created.

Mooladhara: Instinctive in nature (Tamsik). When Bindu falls down to Swadisthana & Mooladhara, it becomes a poison, causing suffering, disease & death.

At Swadisthana, Instant Urge is created for fulfilling the desires and passions. That is why, scriptures advice to adopt certain yogic pattern for lifting the Bindu. Kriya yoga helps to achieve this aspect.

At Mooladhara, the Bindu signifies Instinctive in nature (Tamsik). When Bindu falls down to Swadisthana & Mooladhara, it becomes a poison, causing suffering, disease & death. Probably, because of this reason,

Upanishad indicates the warning that Kriya yoga (Maha Mudra) is a very powerful & the same should be kept secret with care and should not be given to anyone.

5.1.1 Fear of death deteriorate the Human personality

Patanjali has described five Klesha, the hindrances for personality development in worldly as well as in Spiritual life. Among them, Abhinivesha (fear of death) is prominent one. This sustains whenever nuclei (Bindu) remain at three lower chakras especially, at Swadisthana and Mooladhara. The image describes the main characteristics in personality whenever fear of death persists in individual.

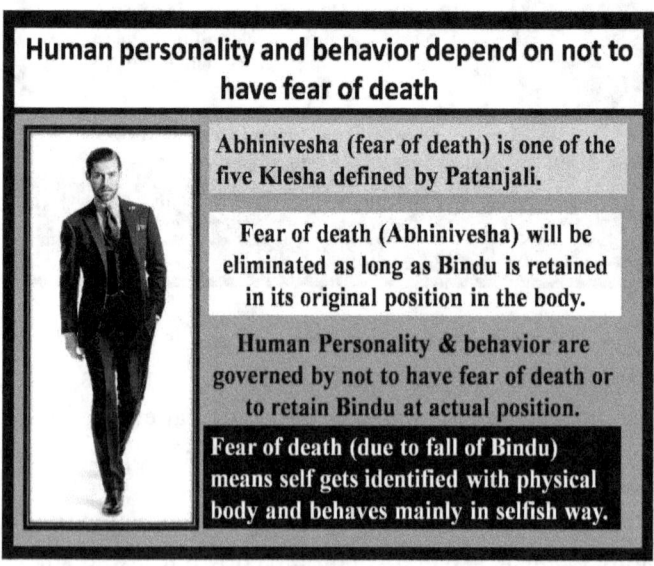

Human personality and behavior depend on not to have fear of death

Abhinivesha (fear of death) is one of the five Klesha defined by Patanjali.

Fear of death (Abhinivesha) will be eliminated as long as Bindu is retained in its original position in the body.

Human Personality & behavior are governed by not to have fear of death or to retain Bindu at actual position.

Fear of death (due to fall of Bindu) means self gets identified with physical body and behaves mainly in selfish way.

Abhinivesha (fear of death) is one of the five Klesha

defined by Patanjali. Fear of death comes as a speed breaker in the path of progressive life journey. Even after certain progress or achievement there will be great hurdles to develop the dynamic personality.

Fear of death (Abhinivesha) will be eliminated as long as Bindu is retained in its original position in the body. Whenever if there is a fall of female characteristics of Bindu at Vishuddhi and Anahata chakra, there will not be complete removal of fear of death but the same will be of minimum order.

Human Personality & behavior (of great people) are governed by not to have fear of death or to retain Bindu at Bindu Visarga. At this position of Bindu, the divinity is retained by a great personality to have Bindu as a launching pad. From there, one can be a very successful person in Worldly life or he or she can rapidly progress in Spiritual life also.

Fear of death (due to fall of Bindu) means self gets identified with physical body and behaves mainly in selfish way. This shows that fear of death is a great hindrance to come out from the gross body and be progressive in subtle and causal body. That is why; the very selfish person will be under the grief of fear of death.

5.2 Merger of Two Bindu (second principle of Kriya yoga)

The process of unifying or sublimating these two Bindu can be achieved easily with the help of Kriya yoga process. By achieving the merger, the people become eligible for getting connected with the supreme reality which in turn provides the freedom from life and death.

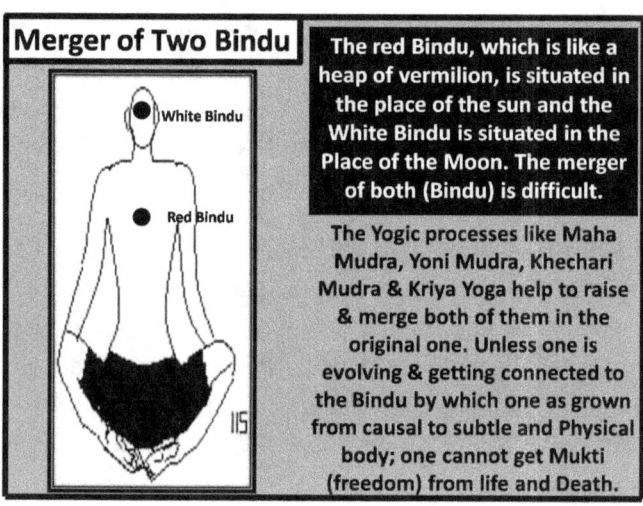

Merger of Two Bindu

White Bindu

Red Bindu

The red Bindu, which is like a heap of vermilion, is situated in the place of the sun and the White Bindu is situated in the Place of the Moon. The merger of both (Bindu) is difficult.

The Yogic processes like Maha Mudra, Yoni Mudra, Khechari Mudra & Kriya Yoga help to raise & merge both of them in the original one. Unless one is evolving & getting connected to the Bindu by which one as grown from causal to subtle and Physical body; one cannot get Mukti (freedom) from life and Death.

The red Bindu, which is like a heap of vermilion, is situated in the place of the sun and the White Bindu is situated in the Place of the Moon. The merger of both (Bindu) is difficult. By practicing Maha Mudra (essential steps like Asana, Pranayama, Bandha and Maha Bheda Mudra) and also by practicing Yoni Mudra (essential steps like closer of 9 gates with the help of bandha and placement of fingers on Gyan Indriya, Pranayama or Inner Kumbhak along with Maha Bheda Mudra) will help to raise the red Bindu at Bindu Visarga and also to merge both of them. Unless one is evolving & getting connected to the Bindu by which one as grown from causal to subtle and Physical body; one cannot get Mukti (freedom) from life and death.

6. FIRST STEP OF KRIYA YOGA

The basic principle of Kriya Yoga is to raise the lower nucleus (having a structure present in most cells, containing the genetic material) at higher Chakra so as to achieve vibrant and dynamic personality in day-to-day life. Further, Kriya Yoga helps to achieve the divine personality which is a stepping stone for progressive and Quantum jump in meditation. In brief, Kriya Yoga helps to have progressive materialistic life as well as to evolve in the field of transcendental domain.

The actual use of Kriya Yoga is to raise the Apana Prana to higher centers and ultimately to establish the unification of lower mental energy (feminine characteristics) with Chandra (at Bindu Visarga) .At start with (during inception), Bindu Visarga is the point for individual to have three bodies creation (Physical, Subtle and Causal body). Till youth hood is achieved, the original Bindu gets divided into two nuclei. One stays weak at Bindu Visarga and other gets shifted to Anahata (sun place) in normal person. However, during youth hood the feminine characteristics of Bindu remains at Swadisthana. If the same is slowly raised to moon (at top back of the head or Bindu Visarga), they get merged or united. This process is achieved by Kriya Yoga Practice easily.

6.1 Complete knowledge of Kriya yoga (Maha Mudra) is essential

Normally, the seekers of Kriya yoga do not get the full knowledge of Kriya yoga. They simply get the demonstration of what they are supposed to do. They are not aware of the aim and objective of Kriya yoga and what Kriya yoga does during the practice. They simply know that the same is advantageous for meditation and healthy life. In absence of complete knowledge of Kriya yoga, there is likelihood of committing some mistakes and get trapped by the harmful effect of Kriya yoga (if not understood and followed properly). The mantra number 65 of Yoga Chudamani Upanishad provides the brief description of Maha Mudra (the first and foremost part of Kriya yoga).

Maha Mudra is the process for purification of Nadi (movement of sun or Moon) & Absorption of Vital Fluid. Kriya Yoga involves all (Asana, Pranayama, Mudra and Bandha). The purification of Nadi is very essential as it provides the basic structure of the subtle body. Unless the same is purified and strengthened, the absorption of vital fluid at different chakra of the body will not be successful. Maha Mudra technique helps in three ways namely i) purification of Nadi ii) uplifting of vital fluid and iii) absorption of the same (vital fluid) in gaseous form at different parts of the body including brain so that all get strengthened.

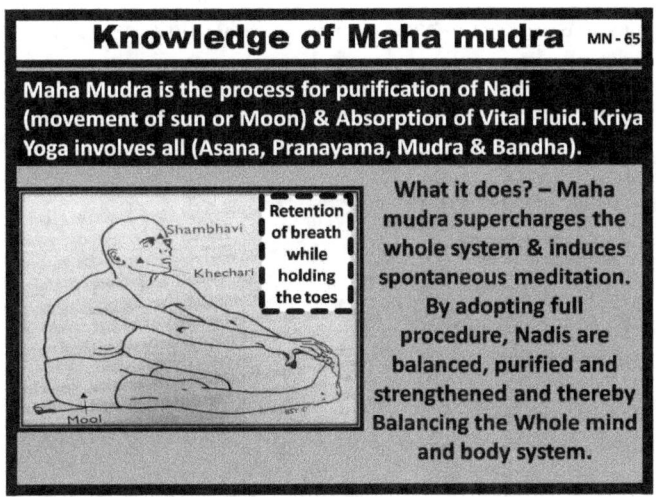

Knowledge of Maha mudra MN-65

Maha Mudra is the process for purification of Nadi (movement of sun or Moon) & Absorption of Vital Fluid. Kriya Yoga involves all (Asana, Pranayama, Mudra & Bandha).

Retention of breath while holding the toes

What it does? – Maha mudra supercharges the whole system & induces spontaneous meditation. By adopting full procedure, Nadis are balanced, purified and strengthened and thereby Balancing the Whole mind and body system.

What it does? – Maha mudra supercharges the whole system & induces spontaneous meditation. By adopting full procedures, Nadis are balanced, purified and strengthened and thereby balancing the Whole mind and body system. The function described above can be achieved easily by following the steps given in Maha Mudra like Asana, Pranayama (including retention of breath or inner Kumbhak), Bandha (for upliftment and retention of Apana prana at higher chakra) and Maha Bheda Mudra (for inducing the effect of vibration in brain) to achieve the inner movement of neurons. In addition, this also helps to make the digestive system stronger and cures all the diseases in day to day life.

6.2 Importance of Kriya Yoga

The importance of Kriya yoga can be visualized in many ways. For instance, Maha Mudra improves the pranic flow as well as the stability of Nucleus (controller of energy and space or Shiva & Shakti) to uplift human consciousness. To have the complete understanding of its importance, the knowledge of Holism (Purnta) of physical, subtle and causal body is to be understood.

Effect of Maha Mudra on Prana and Bindu MN-65

i. The flow of Pranic energy in Sushumna is stimulated & thereby increasing awareness, Inducing clarity of thought & removing nervous depression. ii. Maha Mudra governs the movement of Prana and Bindu in Moon & Sun centre. iii. It prevents Bindu to fall and reverses Bindu even after falling.

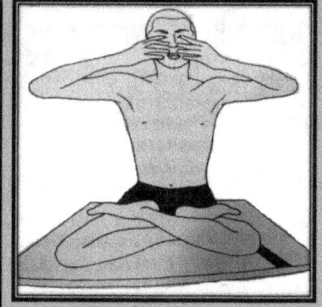

iv. By preserving Bindu from being burnt by sun or passed out through semen and Ovum, the rasas or vital body fluids are reabsorbed.

v. This leads to greater mental and vital power, which can be utilized for regenerating the system or awakening the higher mental faculties

The image describes the importance of Kriya yoga (Maha Mudra) in the following manner:

i. The flow of Pranic energy in Sushumna is stimulated & thereby increasing awareness, inducing clarity of thought & removing nervous depression. This is because, Sushumna is connected to the nervous system and it also contains the path of nuclei (Bindu).

By improving the movement of nuclei (Bindu) in upward chakra, the nervous system is strengthened.

ii. Maha Mudra governs the movement of Prana and Bindu in Moon & Sun centre (top back of the head and Anahata region respectively). When nucleus and prana get synchronized, naturally the third one which is mind also gets synchronized along with prana and nucleus. This way all three get stabilized.

iii. It prevents Bindu to fall and reverses Bindu even after falling. By practicing Maha mudra (Kriya yoga), the prevention is achieved with the help of lifting vital fluid and getting the same spread in the brain region with the help of Maha Bheda Mudra.

iv. By preserving Bindu from being burnt by sun or passed out through semen and Ovum, the Rasas or vital body fluids are reabsorbed. This happens by critically following Moola and Uddiyan Bandha along with retention of inner Kumbhak in the process of Maha Mudra.

v. This (Maha Mudra) leads to greater mental and vital power, which can be utilized for regenerating the system or awakening the higher mental faculties.

6.3 Benefits of Maha Mudra

Maha Mudra provides many benefits like prevention and cure of many contiguous, non contiguous and killer diseases such as cancer, HIV, Swine Flu, Ebola virus etc. It develops the immune capability of an individual and brings out the hidden potentiality of human being. The digestive system of an individual is also improved by Maha Mudra practice; hence the extraction and assimilation of vitamins and minerals present in the food are adequately obtained.

6.3.1 Maha Mudra cures all the diseases

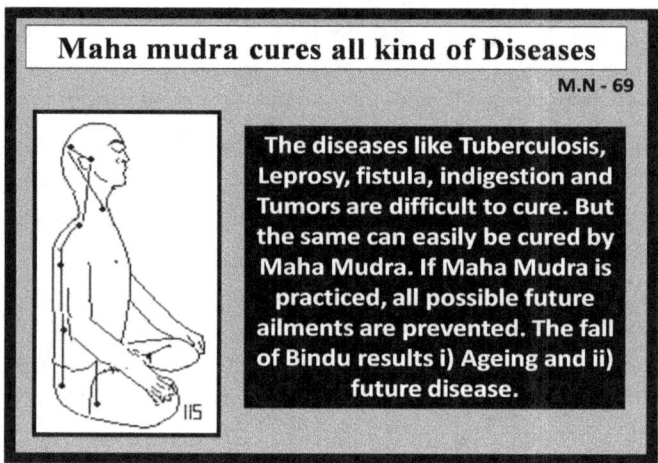

Maha mudra cures all kind of Diseases

M.N - 69

The diseases like Tuberculosis, Leprosy, fistula, indigestion and Tumors are difficult to cure. But the same can easily be cured by Maha Mudra. If Maha Mudra is practiced, all possible future ailments are prevented. The fall of Bindu results i) Ageing and ii) future disease.

The diseases like Tuberculosis, Leprosy, fistula, indigestion and Tumors are difficult to cure. Few centuries ago these diseases where very difficult to get cured and they where curse for the human kind. But the same can easily be cured by Maha Mudra. The seers have observed that the practice of Maha Mudra can cure such kind of diseases. This is because; Apana prana and the position of nuclei (Bindu) get uplifted to work with their healthy characteristics (quality and quantity) at upper chakra.

If Maha Mudra is practiced, all possible future

ailments are prevented. This is because, the fall of Bindu results i) Ageing and ii) future disease. The fall of nuclei (Bindu) at Manipura chakra will enhance the depletion of nectar (Amrit) by burning the same. This means that the nuclei of blood cells will be deprived of basic nutrients which were otherwise supplied from the cosmic (Atma) domain. This will lead to earlier ageing of the people.

The fall of Bindu from Anahata chakra will create imbalance of prana (energy) to fight against the viruses and microbes of the future diseases. When nuclei (Bindu) fall down to Swadisthana, the concerned energy (prana) and space (concerned level of mind) can function with lower characteristics (quality and quantity). This is because; nuclei (Bindu) holds reign of energy and space. The inter linking of energy, space & controller and ruler of their (energy and space) characteristics can be re called for clarity.

6.4 The basis of Maha Mudra to cure diseases

Maha Mudra does three kinds of activities in the system to prevent and cure the chronic diseases. They are i) preventing the fall of nuclei (Bindu) at lower chakra ii) stimulation of pranic energy at higher chakra and iii) fusion of two prana at higher chakra. These activities have been summarized in the image.

It stimulates the Prana in the frontal and Spinal energy circuits from Mooladhara to Bindu Chakra and removes energy blocks from Pranic & Psychic system. Pranic system of energy flow remains in frontal zone and psychic system of energy flow remains in spinal cord. The psychic system of energy flow is controlled by nuclei (Bindu). For stimulation, when Bindu is raised from lower region (in a spinal cord) to higher region, the connected prana or energy is also lifted to higher chakra in the frontal region. This means the Apana prana is getting stimulated to remain in upward direction (Urdhvagati) in the influence of nuclei (Bindu). Without raising the Bindu, there will be blockage in the flow of pranic system. Though the blockage could be removed by other means of Pranayama too, the same is enhancing by uplifting the Bindu.

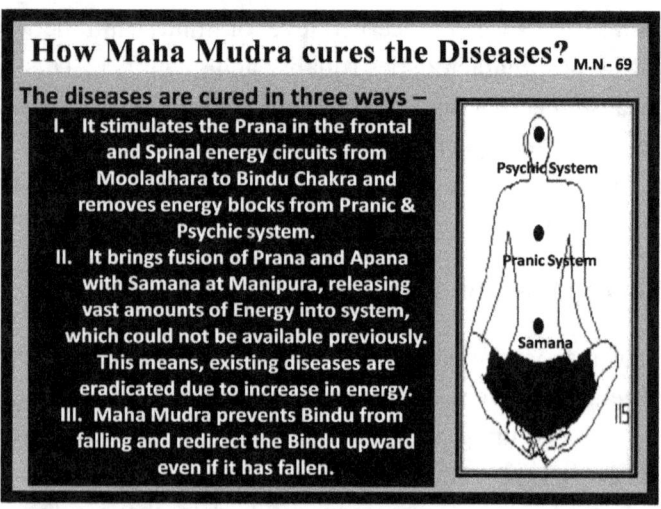

How Maha Mudra cures the Diseases? M.N - 69

The diseases are cured in three ways –

I.   It stimulates the Prana in the frontal and Spinal energy circuits from Mooladhara to Bindu Chakra and removes energy blocks from Pranic & Psychic system.

II. It brings fusion of Prana and Apana with Samana at Manipura, releasing vast amounts of Energy into system, which could not be available previously. This means, existing diseases are eradicated due to increase in energy.

III. Maha Mudra prevents Bindu from falling and redirect the Bindu upward even if it has fallen.

It brings fusion of Prana and Apana with Samana at Manipura, releasing vast amounts of Energy into system, which could not be available previously. This means, existing diseases are eradicated due to increase in energy. When Apana prana is brought up to the region of Manipura chakra (the field of Samana prana) then they get fused under the influence of nuclei (Bindu) in psychic system (in spinal cord). When Apana prana and Samana prana become one, the same retains the vast amount of energy which otherwise was not available. This vast amount of energy eradicates or neutralizes the existing diseases.

Maha Mudra prevents Bindu from falling and redirects the Bindu upward even if it has fallen. The practice of Pranayama, Bandha (Moola and Uddiyan Bandha) and retention of Prana at Agna chakra of Maha Mudra help the nuclei (Bindu) to be retained at higher psychic region. This happens even if nuclei (Bindu) fall down up to Manipura region.

6.5 Maha Mudra improves digestive system

To analysis explains how digestive system is strengthened by Maha Mudra. It clarifies that the practice of Moola bandha, Uddiyan bandha and upliftment of Bindu in psychic channel can enhance the digestive system as well as the spiritual awareness. The image summarizes the same is brief.

By Uddiyan Bandha Samana Prana is increased. Nasikagra mudra and Moola Bandha stimulate Mooladhara chakra and redirect the downward flow of Apana upward to Manipura. In first step, when we go for Moola bandha and Nasikagra mudra the Apana prana moves upward direction from Mooladhara chakra to Manipura chakra. The Samana Prana gets strengthened because of addition of Apana prana at Manipur chakra.

By adopting the Uddiyan bandha the strengthened Samana prana (original Samana prana and added Apana prana) is further increased.

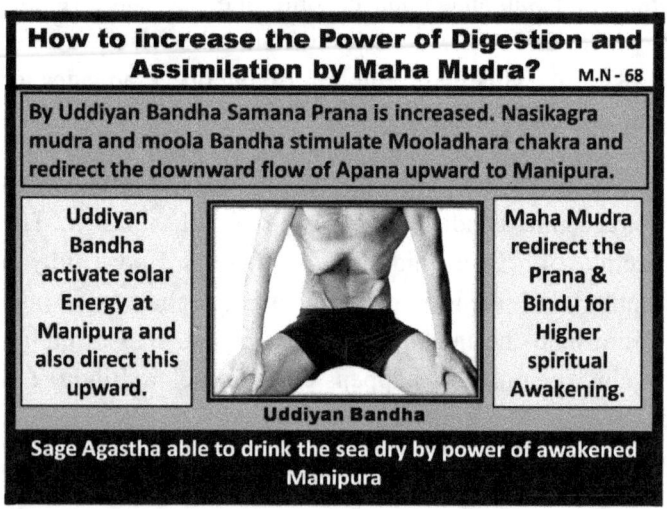

How to increase the Power of Digestion and Assimilation by Maha Mudra? M.N - 68

By Uddiyan Bandha Samana Prana is increased. Nasikagra mudra and moola Bandha stimulate Mooladhara chakra and redirect the downward flow of Apana upward to Manipura.

Uddiyan Bandha activate solar Energy at Manipura and also direct this upward.

Uddiyan Bandha

Maha Mudra redirect the Prana & Bindu for Higher spiritual Awakening.

Sage Agastha able to drink the sea dry by power of awakened Manipura

Uddiyan Bandha activates solar Energy at Manipura and also directs this upward. This is the added advantage of Uddiyan bandha. At this point the solar energy (normally indicated at Anahata region) is strengthened and moved upwards for further unveiling of psychic experiences.

Maha Mudra redirects the Prana & Bindu for Higher spiritual Awakening. The practice of Maha mudra helps to raise Apana prana up to Samana prana region and get them fused.

Further, it helps to uplift the fused prana up to Anahata region to experience the psychic phenomena. This means the practice of Kriya yoga (Maha Mudra)

retains the full control of three Prana (Apana, Samana and Prana) by keeping the integrated prana at higher region of the human system.

Sage Agastha able to drink the sea dry by power of awakened Manipura. The example of sage Agastha indicates that if full control of Manipura region is obtained with the help of Maha mudra or Kriya yoga, the power of digestive system can be increased tremendously and anything & everything can be digested.

6.6 Different utility of Maha Mudra

The steps given in Maha Mudra are linked to have the beneficial effect on i) physical level ii) vital force (prana) level iii) psychological dimension and iv) psychic dimension.

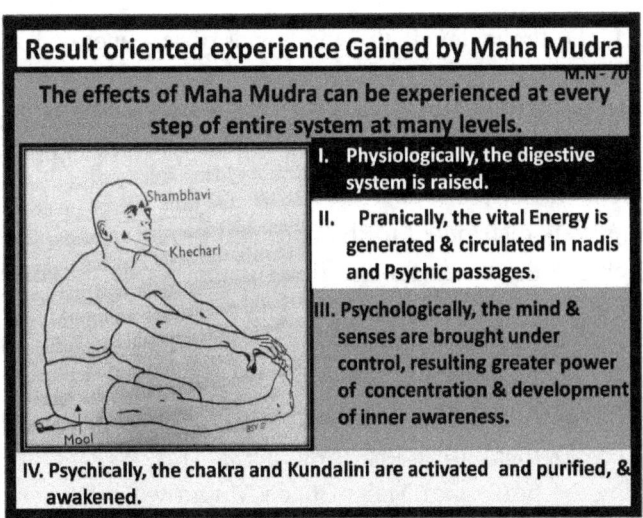

Result oriented experience Gained by Maha Mudra

The effects of Maha Mudra can be experienced at every step of entire system at many levels.

I. Physiologically, the digestive system is raised.

II. Pranically, the vital Energy is generated & circulated in nadis and Psychic passages.

III. Psychologically, the mind & senses are brought under control, resulting greater power of concentration & development of inner awareness.

IV. Psychically, the chakra and Kundalini are activated and purified, & awakened.

There are major five steps followed in Maha Mudra. The process of Asana and Pranayama (in Maha Mudra) helps to strengthen the physical dimensions so as to Samana prana at digestive system is raised. Likewise, other benefits are also linked. The image summarizes the benefits at different levels.

The image describes the effects of Maha Mudra at different steps and the same can be experienced if Maha Mudra is followed correctly. The benefits have been summarized and they are as follows:

I. Physiologically, the digestive system is raised. This happens as the Apana prana, which seems to be energy drainer because of its existence at lower chakra, is raised and merged with Samana prana. Because of this, digestive system becomes stronger and physically we enjoy the sound health.

II. At Prana level, the vital energy is generated & circulated in nadis and Psychic passages. This is achieved with the help of Moola and Uddiyan bandha where the bandha helps to retain the vital fluid at higher centers. In turn the distribution of vital fluid at higher center gets distributed to the nadi and psychic passages; which are the bases for the flow of the pranic (energy) system.

III. Psychologically, the mind & senses are brought under control, resulting greater power of concentration & development of inner awareness. This is achieved during the process of Maha Bheda Mudra when the vital fluid brought from the down is forcibly circulated in the solid mass of the brain. Maha Bheda Mudra helps to activate the protein polymer (grey colored solid mass) to provide the ways for the function of neurons. This process can help the psychologist to cure the chronic mental cases as central zone of the brain (where motor and sensory organs exist) becomes synchronized. In addition, it also helps the practitioner of meditation to concentrate and find the expansion of inner awareness.

IV. Psychically, the chakra and Kundalini are activated and purified & awakened. This can be obtained as the steps of Asana, Pranayama (including inner and outer Kumbhak), bandha (Moola and Uddiyan) and Maha Bheda Pranayama are followed in Kriya yoga. The whole process in turn, activates the chakra existed in frontal zone and purifies the same. In the long run the path of Kundalini is also activated and purified.

6.7 Beneficial aspects of Maha Mudra for psychologist

After inception, there is a growth of causal, subtle and physical body in mother's womb and also outside till we achieve the youth hood. During the process the essence or nuclei (Bindu) coming from almighty becomes two and they are situated at top back of the head and in the region of heart. For male gender nuclei at top back of the head is dominating whereas for female gender nuclei at heart region (rajas or red) is dominating. They represent the higher and lower mind and have many effects on human mind which is the field of a psychologist. That is why, the structure of the brain has to be understood where Kriya yoga (Maha Mudra) helps a lot to streamline the flow of inner potential.

While manifestation progressive transformation from causal to subtle and further to gross body, the division of energy and space from the original nucleus is bound to happen for the stability of higher and lower mind. The lower mind consisting main energy (prana) to provide functional requirement of strength for the function of senses (Karma Indriya and Gyan Indriya). The higher mental energy is responsible for motor control of the brain. The function of lower mind and higher mind (energy required for sense organs and control of the autonomous nervous system) is mainly situated in middle part of the brain.

It is interesting to note that the functional aspects of the brain can be divided into three segments like frontal brain, middle brain and rear brain. The frontal brain is responsible for thinking, ethics and creative aspects of the brain. The middle brain consists of motor and sensory control whereas rear brain will sum up (conclusive) aspects of the activity. The image describes the brief a structure and function of the brain.

The image clearly indicates that the psychological problem becomes more serious when there are discrepancies in functional aspects of motor and sensory organs. Middle part of the brain is responsible for having mismatch of psychic energy and results the psychological problems. If any system or method can help to synchronize the activity of motor and sensory organs (situated at middle part of the brain), the same is welcomed. The Indian seer has visualized a system known as Kriya yoga with the help of Maha Mudra to achieve the harmoniously balanced mind even after the mismatch of psychic forces. The analysis shows the beneficial effect of Kriya yoga on psychological problems.

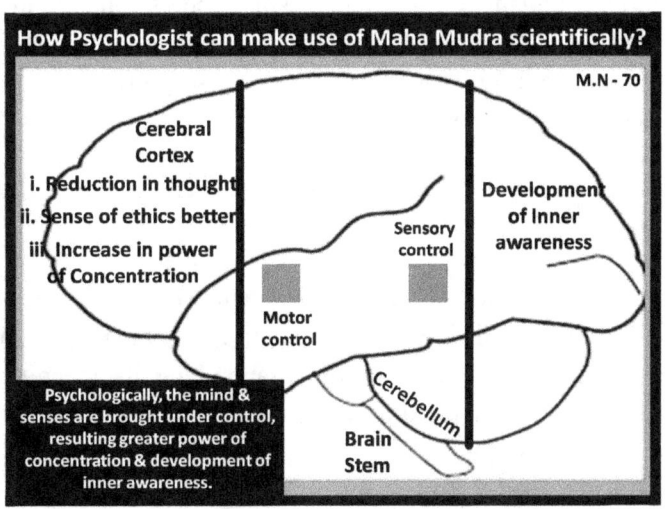

How Psychologist can make use of Maha Mudra scientifically?

M.N - 70

Cerebral Cortex
i. Reduction in thought
ii. Sense of ethics better
iii. Increase in power of Concentration

Development of Inner awareness

Sensory control

Motor control

Psychologically, the mind & senses are brought under control, resulting greater power of concentration & development of inner awareness.

Cerebellum

Brain Stem

Psychologically, in the process of Kriya yoga, the mind & senses are brought under control resulting greater power of concentration & development of inner awareness. During psychological problems the mind is fluctuating very rapidly and the same can generates about more than fifty thousand thoughts per day. The energy is rapidly drained and patient cannot concentrate on any subject. In this way he or she cannot remain fully aware of what one is doing.

The concentration and awareness is achieved during the process of Maha Bheda Mudra when the vital fluid brought from the down is forcibly circulated in the solid mass of the brain. Maha Bheda Mudra helps to activate the protein polymer (grey colored solid mass) to provide the ways for the function of neurons. When the vital fluid is spread forcibly in the solid mass of the brain, the process of strengthening the weaker organs of the brain starts and mismatch is reduced. This process can help the psychologist to cure the chronic mental cases as central zone of the brain (where motor and sensory organs exist) becomes synchronized.

6.8 Why Maha Mudra should be kept secret with care?

Mantra number 70 states that Maha Mudra should be kept secret with care and it should not be taught to anyone. The image reads the Mantra and its meaning signifies the beneficial aspects as well as the reasons for keeping the same secretly.

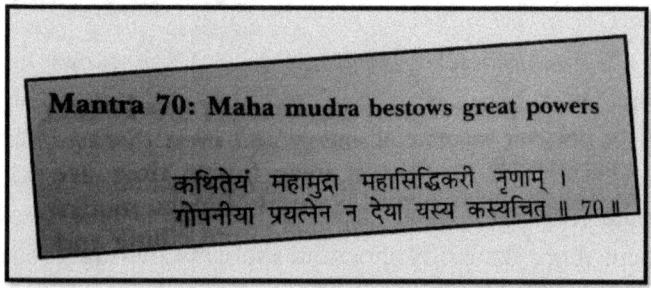

Mantra 70: Maha mudra bestows great powers

कथितेयं महामुद्रा महासिद्धिकरी नृणाम् ।
गोपनीया प्रयत्नेन न देया यस्य कस्यचित् ॥ 70 ॥

However, Maha Mudra bestows great power to those who are practicing correctly. Maha Mudra bestows the Power for curing diseases. This happens because inner organs like Kidney, Pancreas, Spleen, Bladder, Lungs get full exposure of fresh oxygen for cleansing and in turn they become strengthened. Maha Mudra also provides the great power to digestive system. This is possible as Apana Prana (energy drainer) gets uplifted and gets united with Samana Prana (the energy responsible for digestion). This way, Samana Prana becomes very strong. By knowing the great power bestowed by Kriya yoga, why then the same should be kept secret with care?

Now a days (In the age of Internet), Kriya Yoga is taught through Mail, Chat, Video call, Webinar, Wikipedia, Video conferencing and also through massive work shop. Because of its popularity, seeker does not verify the authentic evolution of the master (due to fast life style) and learns the steps of Kriya Yoga (Maha mudra and Yoni Mudra) without knowing its harm, if not practiced correctly. That is why, earlier master (Guru) used to be present while performing Kriya Yoga at least for some times. To understand the consequences (if Kriya Yoga is not done properly), the research on the Purpose of Kriya Yoga and Basic principle behind it (Kriya Yoga) have to be carried out rigorously.

The image describes that the importance of anything is lost when discussed publically. The other factors which could probably be harmful to the people (who are not perfectly doing or who are not eligible to have Kriya yoga) are also summarized in the image.

When the practice of great power is discussed publically, it loses its potential. In Hatha Yoga

Pradeepika it states that Yogis who wish to attain perfection keep the practice highly secret. In order to be powerful, it must be kept secret as reveled once will be Powerless. This is because, while reveling, some of the methods might be lost if the teacher is not fully matured. Even the matured practitioner can do the mistakes if they do not know the principle and purpose of Kriya yoga.

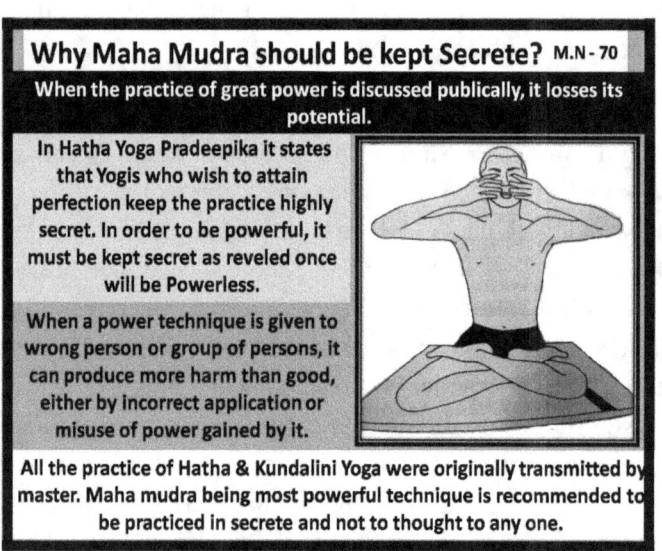

Why Maha Mudra should be kept Secrete? M.N-70

When the practice of great power is discussed publically, it losses its potential.

In Hatha Yoga Pradeepika it states that Yogis who wish to attain perfection keep the practice highly secret. In order to be powerful, it must be kept secret as reveled once will be Powerless.

When a power technique is given to wrong person or group of persons, it can produce more harm than good, either by incorrect application or misuse of power gained by it.

All the practice of Hatha & Kundalini Yoga were originally transmitted by master. Maha mudra being most powerful technique is recommended to be practiced in secrete and not to thought to any one.

When a power technique is given to wrong person or group of persons, it can produce more harm than good, either by incorrect application or misuse of power gained by it. That is why the full science of Kriya yoga should be understood before taking of this course.

All the practice of Hatha & Kundalini Yoga was originally transmitted by master. Maha mudra being most powerful technique is recommended to be practiced in secrete and not to thought to anyone. This is because, the equivalent other proven practices are available in Astang yoga where the mistakes carried out will not yield the greater harm.

Kriya Yoga (with the help of Maha Mudra) performed with perfection, the same yields Siddhi. The Siddhi achieved by Kriya Yoga is comprised of certain similar points likely to obtain through Kundalini Yoga. If Sadhaka of Kriya yoga is not fully matured, he or she would like to misuse the great power of Kriya Yoga against the society. Another reason for keeping this Yoga very secret with care could be because of mistakes likely to be carried out or processes involved in Kriya yoga are not performed properly.

The mantra also states that at Mooladhara, the Bindu signifies Instinctive in nature (Tamsik). When Bindu falls down to Swadisthana & Mooladhara, it becomes a poison, causing suffering, disease & death. Probably, because of this reason, Upanishad indicates the warning that Kriya yoga (Maha Mudra) is a very powerful & the same should be kept secret with care and should not be given to anyone.

■

7. SECOND STEP OF KRIYA YOGA (SHANMUKHI OR YONI MUDRA)

Shanmukhi mudra is another important aspect of Kriya Yoga to have sustainable stability of Apana Prana and vital fluid at higher Chakra by adopting Asana, Pranayama, Bandha and Mudra position effectively. The important aspect of Yoni Mudra is to be noted. One among them is the closure of nine gates through which energy leaks out. In this Mudra, the nine gates (two ears, two eyes, two nostrils, mouth, genital organ and solid excretory) are to be kept closure while inhalation and retention. During Maha Bheda Mudra (essential for activation of neurons), three gates (mouth and two nostrils) are only opened and others remain closed.

The main difference between Maha Mudra and Yoni Mudra is to be analyzed. In case of Maha mudra, during inhalation main attention is given on vital fluid along with prana (energy). That process is very effective especially for digestive system and for the cure of diseases. In Yoni mudra process, attention is given mainly on lifting of Apana prana and adopting the process to retain the same (Apana prana) at higher chakra. The retention is achieved by closure of nine gates; which is very important. Otherwise, the process of Yoni mudra (Shanmukhi mudra) is not effective.

7.1 Movement of prana during Yoni Mudra

The nuclei (Bindu) are the regulator and controller of prana (energy) and also Chetana (space). If Bindu falls down, there is likelihood of falling of Bindu at lower centers. This method (Yoni Mudra) ensures that the regulator & controller of prana and Chetana (energy and space) are kept at higher centers by closure of nine openings of the energy falls.

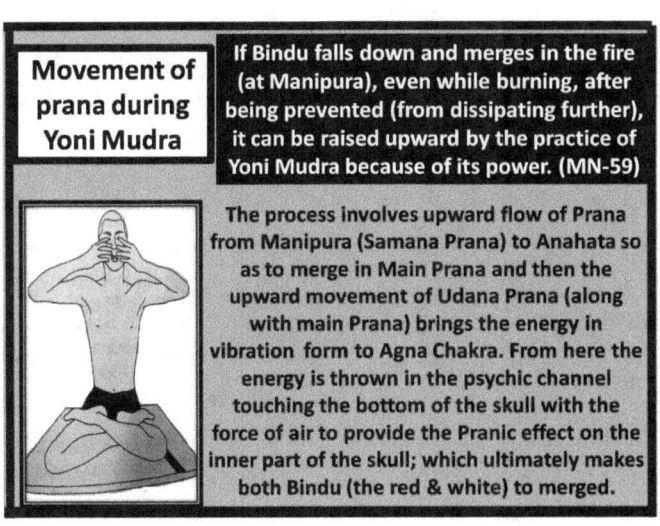

Movement of prana during Yoni Mudra

If Bindu falls down and merges in the fire (at Manipura), even while burning, after being prevented (from dissipating further), it can be raised upward by the practice of Yoni Mudra because of its power. (MN-59)

The process involves upward flow of Prana from Manipura (Samana Prana) to Anahata so as to merge in Main Prana and then the upward movement of Udana Prana (along with main Prana) brings the energy in vibration form to Agna Chakra. From here the energy is thrown in the psychic channel touching the bottom of the skull with the force of air to provide the Pranic effect on the inner part of the skull; which ultimately makes both Bindu (the red & white) to merged.

If Bindu falls down and merges in the fire (at Manipura), even while burning, after being prevented (from dissipating further), it can be raised upward by the practice of Yoni Mudra because of its power. Normally, Rajas Bindu remains at Anahata chakra for the practitioner of Kriya yoga, especially in the case of female. In case of male the same may like to fall down at Manipura chakra where it gets burnt. In day to day activity, when there is a possibility to fall the Bindu at Manipura chakra, the same can be prevented from burning by raising it at higher chakra. This is achieved easily with the help of Yoni mudra.

The process involves upward flow of Prana from Manipura (Samana Prana) to Anahata so as to merge in Main Prana and then the upward movement of Udana Prana (along with main Prana) brings the energy in vibration form to Agna Chakra. From here the energy is thrown in the psychic channel touching the bottom of the skull with the force of air to provide the Pranic effect on the inner part of the skull; which ultimately makes both Bindu (the red & white) to merged.

The successive lifting of Apana prana to merge with Samana prana and then to become Maha prana and ultimately to unite with Udana prana helps a lot to reach the pituitary gland (Agna chakra) in a sustainable form. This is required for the people who are the Spiritual seeker. After reaching its (pranic energy) up to maximum strength the utility of the same is obtained by forcing it with the help of external flow of air (by making sound eee....) at lower portion of the skull (brain).

The forcible integration of Maha prana in the skull

helps to activate the grey mass of the brain. To lose the protein polymer structure of the brain, this part of Maha Bheda Mudra helps a lot and makes the red Bindu (Rajas Bindu, also known as lower mind)   to merge with white Bindu at Bindu Visarga (top back of the head). When merger is over then Sadhaka becomes divine to take a quantum jump in the domain of transcendental body through Turiya.

7.2 Yoni Mudra invokes the power of creation

Khechari mudra is the best possible solution for retaining the Bindu at Bindu Visarga. But its perfection is very difficult.

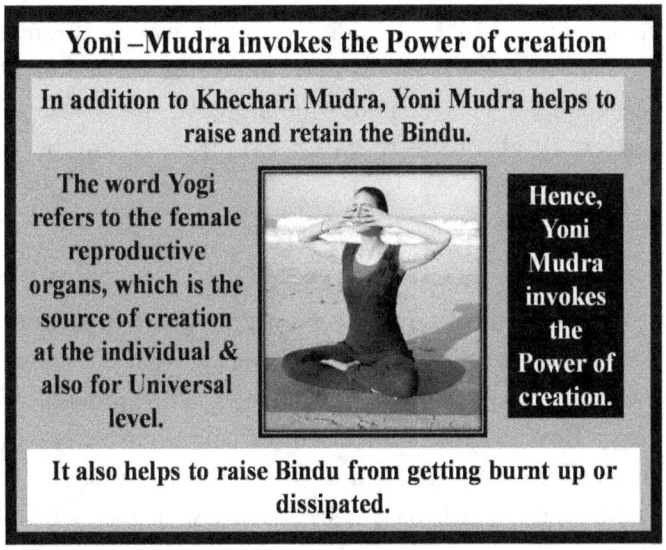

Yoni –Mudra invokes the Power of creation

In addition to Khechari Mudra, Yoni Mudra helps to raise and retain the Bindu.

The word Yogi refers to the female reproductive organs, which is the source of creation at the individual & also for Universal level.

Hence, Yoni Mudra invokes the Power of creation.

It also helps to raise Bindu from getting burnt up or dissipated.

That is why; Indian seers have found another mudra known as Yoni mudra which raises the red Bindu (nuclei) at top back of the head to retain and merge with white Bindu. This mudra also prevents the burning of red Bindu at Manipura chakra if practiced without committing any mistake.

The image describes that the Khechari Mudra & Yoni Mudra help to raise and retain the Bindu. That is why; this mudra is practiced many times in Kriya yoga to achieve the perfection. Main attention is drawn about the closure of nine openings of the senses to the practitioner of Kriya yoga. Is this is not followed strictly, the full benefits of Kriya yoga is not obtained.

The word Yogi refers to the female reproductive organs, which is the source of creation at the individual & also for Universal level. When the concept of Bindu (nuclei) is analyzed, the Yoni is also known as Hiranya Garbha where the creation starts at cosmic as well as in physical level. Hence, Yoni Mudra invokes the Power of creation. It also helps to raise Bindu from getting burnt up or dissipated.

7.3 Process of Yoni Mudra

The main attention is given on Pratyahara process of Astang yoga when withdrawal of energy from the senses is carried out. If this is not done, further process of energy flow in inward direction (or being introvert) will not be successful. The next step is to pay the attention at lower Bindu which has to be known with the help of Tanmatra or the aptitude of lower mind. Even if the position of lower Bindu is not known, the seeker of Kriya yoga need not to worry ; but be strict to raise Apana prana up to Anahata chakra (the region of main prana) and merged both of them so that the lower Bindu (nuclei) is retained at Anahata center. Finally to lift the red or rajas Bindu from Anahata to top back of the head, further lifting of lower Bindu is raised up to Agna chakra. Next step is to be taken for merger of the lower or rajas Bindu with white Bindu with the help of Maha Bheda Mudra. During this process, the mind should be focused at top back of the head.

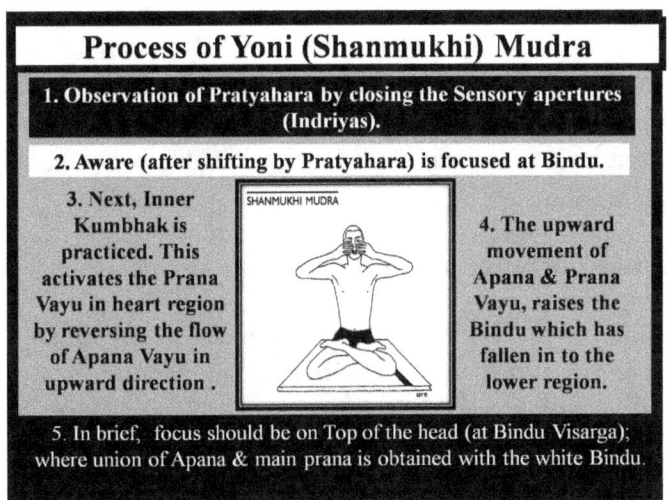

Process of Yoni (Shanmukhi) Mudra

1. Observation of Pratyahara by closing the Sensory apertures (Indriyas).

2. Aware (after shifting by Pratyahara) is focused at Bindu.

3. Next, Inner Kumbhak is practiced. This activates the Prana Vayu in heart region by reversing the flow of Apana Vayu in upward direction .

SHANMUKHI MUDRA

4. The upward movement of Apana & Prana Vayu, raises the Bindu which has fallen in to the lower region.

5. In brief, focus should be on Top of the head (at Bindu Visarga); where union of Apana & main prana is obtained with the white Bindu.

The process of Yoni mudra has been summarized in brief. The image describes the following:

1. Observation of Pratyahara by closing the Sensory apertures (Indriyas). This is necessary step of Astang yoga otherwise mind will not be introvert.

2. Aware (after shifting by Pratyahara) is focused at Red Bindu (situated at Anahata region). This is necessary to locate the red or rajas Bindu at Anahata

region by raising and merging the Apana prana with main Prana.

3. Next, Inner Kumbhak is practiced. This activates the Prana Vayu in heart region by reversing the flow of Apana Vayu in upward direction.

4. The upward movement of Apana & Prana Vayu raises the Bindu which has fallen in to the lower region.

5. Further, the same is lifted up to Agna chakra and allow flowing in the path of psychic tunnel. In brief, focus should be on Top of the head (at Bindu Visarga); where union of Apana & main prana is obtained with the white Bindu.

7.4 Importance of Yoni Mudra

Normally, even for the practitioner of Kriya yoga there is a probable fall of Bindu (main anchor point of energy and space) up to Manipura chakra; where the same gets burnt.

It is important to note that fall of Bindu and get burnt at Manipura chakra will be a great loss to retain a good health and personality. During this process (burning of Bindu), the control of energy (prana) and space (lower mind) is lost and there is likelihood of further fall of energy and space at Swadisthana and Mooladhara region.

That is why Yoni mudra is important to retain and also to raise the Bindu up to top back of the mind. At this point there is a creation of divine platform which works as the source of acceleration during meditation.

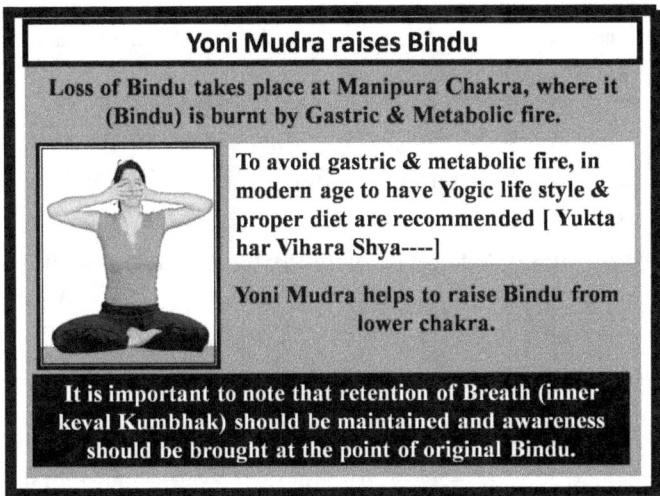

Yoni Mudra raises Bindu

Loss of Bindu takes place at Manipura Chakra, where it (Bindu) is burnt by Gastric & Metabolic fire.

To avoid gastric & metabolic fire, in modern age to have Yogic life style & proper diet are recommended [Yukta har Vihara Shya----]

Yoni Mudra helps to raise Bindu from lower chakra.

It is important to note that retention of Breath (inner keval Kumbhak) should be maintained and awareness should be brought at the point of original Bindu.

The image describes in brief the importance of Yoni Mudra. They are i) Loss of Bindu takes place at Manipura Chakra, where it (Bindu) is burnt by Gastric & Metabolic fire. The Manipura chakra is the point where digestive system works. It is but natural to have imbalance of gastro intestinal problem which is in the form of heat. This heat is responsible for burning up the red or rajas Bindu (lower mind responsible for anchoring energy and space).

ii) To avoid gastric & metabolic fire, in modern age to have Yogic life style & proper diet are recommended [Yukta har Vihara Shya----]. Though yogic life style is helpful to reduce the gastric & metabolic fire but Yoni mudra is more powerful to minimize or eliminate the same.

iii) Yoni Mudra helps to raise Bindu from lower chakra. This is obtained with the help of Pratyahara by closure of nine gates and retention of Maha prana and Apana prana at higher region.

iv) It is important to note that retention of Breath (inner Keval Kumbhak) should be maintained and awareness should be brought at the point of original Bindu. This means the original lower Bindu is presumed to be at Anahata region. Even if it falls down, by raising Apana prana and merging it with main prana will lift up the lower Bindu up to Anahata region.

The second part of Kriya yoga emphasizes this mudra and instruct the seeker to practice Yoni mudra many times in a day. This is because; its benefits and importance are very helpful for practitioner of meditation.

7.4.1 Why Kumbhak is advised in Yoni Mudra?

The basis of Yoni mudra is to have closure of nine gates (the point of outer flow of energy) and retention of breath (Kumbhak) while raising and merging the Apana prana. This is because; the flow of breath has got direct relation with the flow of Bindu. If after raising Apana prana at higher chakra the flow of breath is not retained, there is likelihood of fall of Apana prana and Bindu (nuclei). That is why; second important factor in Yoni mudra is to have retention of breath (Kumbhak).

The image describes the importance of Kumbhak in Yoni mudra. It correlates the flow of breath along with flow of Bindu (anchor point of energy and space). This is because; there is vital connection between the breath & falling of Bindu. This means, Bindu moves along with Breath.

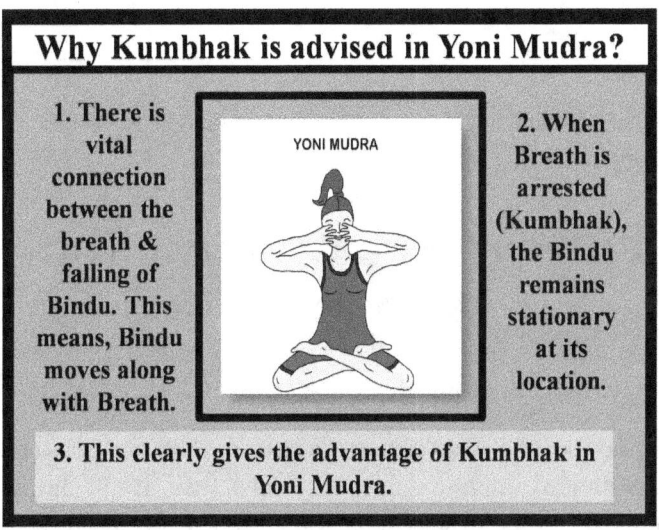

Why Kumbhak is advised in Yoni Mudra?

1. There is vital connection between the breath & falling of Bindu. This means, Bindu moves along with Breath.

YONI MUDRA

2. When Breath is arrested (Kumbhak), the Bindu remains stationary at its location.

3. This clearly gives the advantage of Kumbhak in Yoni Mudra.

This indicates that there should be a methodology to arrest the breath so that the flow (especially downward flow) of Bindu is arrested. When Breath is arrested (Kumbhak), the Bindu remains stationary at its location.

During inner Kumbhak the prana becomes further energized. That is why; many yogic practices follow the inner Kumbhak as Energization process. This is also followed in Yogada Satsang. By Energization of main prana, we achieve the whole some effect of prana (energy); which in turn raise the anchor point (Bindu) as well as Chitta (space) of an individual. This clearly gives the advantage of Kumbhak in Yoni Mudra.

8. IMPORTANCE OF KRIYA YOGA FOR SCIENTISTS

Based on the experience gained in Kriya yoga and Meditation, author strongly feels that if Scientists practice Kriya Yoga (Steps suggested in the book with all cares) can be able to unite and sublimate the lower mind with higher mind. By sublimation, they will be in a position to dive the unknown (Mystic) world, where knowledge and Bliss are available. Sublimation of Lower and higher mind is defined in Upanishad as merging of Shakti (Lower mind) with Shiva (Higher mind). When union happens, the individual becomes Divine and ready to enter in Unknown domain. This domain (unknown or transcendental or the domain of supreme reality) consists of all kinds of knowledge and bliss. The scientist will be in a position to travel in this domain and can be able to invent the conceptual theme either by getting intuition or by direct exposure. This kind of experiment can be exercised as this does not cost anything in respect of time and money.

8.1 Glimpse of human brain

The primitive brain determines our drives mainly for hunger, thirst and reproduction. In case of human being, the outer cell of the brain tissue has mushroomed around the core. This outer shell is the thinking brain. The nervous of the brain is divided in two domains. One is connected to central nervous system and other one is connected to peripheral nerves which are away from the CNS.

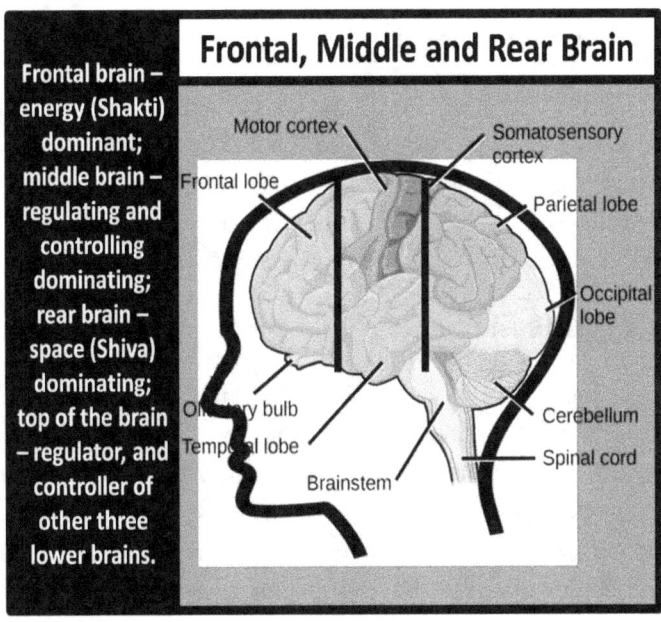

The human brain can be represented in three parts such as i) frontal brain, ii) middle brain and iii) rear (back) brain. Frontal brain contained in cerebral cortex where individual characteristics like animal instinct, urges and rationality exists. This part of the brain exhibit the character of an individual.

Middle brain mainly consists of motor and sensory path, in addition to thalamus and hypothalamus gland. Sensory path receives the information from the body through a spinal cord to brain and motor path send the message from the brain to the body. In case of rear (back) brain, brain stem and its accessories exist. Rear brain is situated in cerebellum cortex. The major important functions have been summarized.

8.2 Function of main parts of brain

Core function, Autonomic nervous system and Somatic nervous system (CAS) is the primitive brain which determines our drives for hunger, thirst & reproduction and also produces the drive for respiratory, digestive and the movement of hands & legs generally.

8.2.1 Brain stem

In the core, brain stem exists. Function of brain stem is to have the control on respiratory and circulatory system along with alarming. The injury of lower part of brain stem (the Pons and Medulla) results in death, as the centers which control respiration, the heart functions and BP are connected here. The brain stem also contains a complex network of brain cells and fibers which runs through its entire length.

The brain cells and fibers receive all the sensations here, and messages pass to the rest of the brain and works like alarm system. For example, if there is a fire, sensation (smell) passes through the alerting network, and thence to the rest of the brain, so that action is taken.

Above the brainstem lies the cerebellum or little brain. It (cerebellum) receives information about movement both from the higher centers (planners) and from the muscles (executers), so that changes can be made. This is important to achieve balance. Thus the cerebellum can be expected to be working very efficiently in a circus trapeze artiste, 'who walks the tight rope'. The cerebellum also plays a role in speech and walking.

8.2.2 Thalamus and Hypothalamus

The thalamus passes all incoming and outgoing information. The hypothalamus lies below the thalamus, it is important for feeling of hunger and thirst as well as to stop them.

The endocrine glands (ductless glands) are pituitary, thyroid; adrenals, pancreas, reproductive glands and their secretions are regulated by hypothalamus. It also controls the ANS (Autonomic Nervous System).

Hypothalamus is also concerned for emotional responses such as pleasure, pain, and rage. Biological clock is also regulated by hypothalamus. Sleep and memory are the two important functions of hypothalamus.

8.2.3 Autonomic Nervous System

Autonomic Nervous System functions like beating of the heart and digestion of food (which is not in our will). It is situated in the brain stem, spinal cord, periphery of nervous system. ANS is controlled by hypothalamus. The ANS has two divisions such as i) the Sympathetic Nervous System (SNS) and ii) Parasympathetic Nervous System (PSNS). PSNS arises from brain stem and the sacral portion of the spinal cord. SNS arises from the thoracic and lumbar parts. In addition, Somatic nervous system functions like walking, moving our hands etc (which is in our will).

8.2.4 Cerebral cortex

Cerebral cortex is responsible for complex functions such as reasoning, creativity and anticipation. There are two cerebral hemispheres known as left hemisphere and right hemisphere. Frontal cortex is the part of the brain which lies behind the forehead. It has been described as the character cortex. The parietal cortex is concerned with putting together information.

8.2.5 Spinal cord

Spinal cord has four parts such as cervical, thoracic, lumbar and sacral portion. Vertebrae offer the protection to the spinal cord which lies within it. The spinal cord is concerned with transmitting sensations (pain, temperature) from the body to the brain. This is called the sensory pathway. The message from the brain to the body comes through motor pathway. The different parts of the spinal cord can also communicate with one another as they are integral part. In some cases, where our responses are very quick and automatic, the spinal cord decides on its own, what has to be done?

8.3 The Blood supply to the brain

Blood supply to the brain is an important factor to understand the major function of brain. Within 5 to 10 seconds of total stoppage of blood supply to the brain, a person loses consciousness, within 2 minutes all the energy stores are used up and the brain death occurs.

It is very interesting to note that the brain makes up about 2% of the body weight- the blood flow/ min is about 15% of the output from the heart. (The average adult brain weighs about 1400 gm). Thus the brain has a blood supply of about 750- 1000 ml/ min. This blood supply remains constant during various conditions, such as exercise and sleep. Probably the most important factor which can make the blood vessels to the brain dilate (become wider) is carbon dioxide. This gas is produced whenever cells are active. Hence when cells are active the carbon dioxide which is produced increases the blood supply automatically.

In addition to blood supply to the brain, the brain also has another fluid, which is clear and transparent. The Cerebro Spinal Fluid (CSF) is formed from the blood. It is present in spaces (ventricles) within the brain. It also present around the brain, between layers of tissue wrapped around the brain. Thus the CSF acts as a 'water cushion'. Normal brain can highly be developed by means of yogic practice so that the scientist will be able to discover the new scientific concepts for utility of human kind.

8.4 Need of vibrant brain

The Scientist having normal brain can also discover some scientific concepts provided they have will power and also the great power of concentration. This is because, both together will uplift their lower mind (which every one posses) to the higher energy centre of the body. The fluctuation of lower mind with low energy can be experienced with an example. For instance, the scientists who do not want to take the risk while formulating the concept, mathematical model and doing some experiment, they would like to follow the safer method and finally will not get the success. This is like a chick (tender bird) in the shell of an egg. It will not prefer to come out from the hard shell as there will be sufficient protection to rest inside the shell where female bird will also take care of the chick. Unless the elder bird will push the chick to fly in the open sky, the chick will never realize the risk factor connected with fly and discover the rest of the world. Scientist of moody nature may find this kind of consequences in the long run.

The other hurdles for the scientists might come in the way about their strong likes and dislikes concerned with people, food, places and environments. This kind of aptitude will anchor the lower mind along with lower energy at Swadisthana chakra which is the centre of Apana prana (an element to drain the normal energy of human system). Hence scientists may take this as the yardstick to visualize the position of their own lower mind.

Emotional is next factor which come as a hurdle for uplifting the lower mind for anyone including the scientists. At this juncture, people will be more moody under negative emotion and their own whole plan will get burnt up in the fire of their being reactive, rejective and grumbling in nature. Next hurdle for the scientist (or any one) for lifting the lower mind is their ego. Unless they know the art of surrendering to their work related to scientific discovery, they may not get success. These hurdles are the outcome of basic nature of scientists which comes from the birth. But the same can be overcome with the help of certain yogic techniques like Kriya yoga and they can achieve the vibrant brain by lifting their lower mind.

8.4.1 How normal brain can be turned into vibrant brain?

Normal brain consists of all the possibilities to explore the hidden potential of divinity (super human being). The question arises, how this could be achieved? Swami Vivekananda has summarized four paths of yoga which can yield the desired result.

They are i) Karma yoga (the path of action) ii) Bhakti yoga (the path of devotion) iii) Gyan yoga (the path of knowledge) and iv) Raj yoga (the path of mind and emotion culture). The brain (mind) can be made vibrant easily with the help of Raj yoga.

8.4.2 The union of two minds is the gateway of vibrant brain

The image describes how Kriya yoga takes care of energy (Shakti) concerned with frontal part of the brain and makes the same equal to the space (Shiva) concerned with rear part of the brain. When both energy (Shakti) and space (Shiva) are equal, the third element consciousness (Brahm) comes into picture for achieving holistic approach. This indicates that merging of the energy and space or Shiva and Shakti evolves the consciousness or Brahm which provides the ability to know the unknown in the Universe.

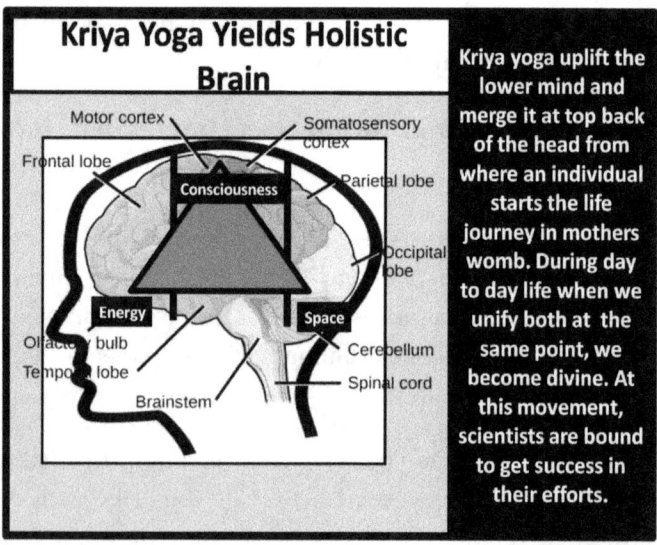

Kriya yoga uplift the lower mind and merge it at top back of the head, from where an individual starts the life journey in mother's womb. This concept is dealt in yoga and the same is known as Bindu (nuclei). This Bindu gets divided into two parts and they are called higher mind (white Bindu) and lower mind (red Bindu). In the life journeys the lower mind having tendency to flow at lower centers (chakra) of the body.

If fall of Bindu (lower mind) continues, our life becomes boredom and miserable. Under this circumstance, the people will not get the success and they may achieve the condition of hopelessness and helplessness.

During day to day life when we unify both at the same point, we become divine. This means the people can achieve a platform after merging the two from there they may plan, organize, lead and control their activities to get success. That is why; this point is the stepping stone for the scientist to achieve the success in their efforts.

8.5 What scientists achieve from Kriya yoga?

Kriya yoga provides very good digestive system and prepare the scientist free from any kind of diseases (claimed by MN- 70 of Yoga Chudamani Upanishad).

This is not philosophical statement by mantra, but the same can be examined by analyzing the purification and activation of three major glands in the brain. The Kriya yoga improves the functional aspects of these glands and provides the desired results. They have been analyzed in detailed.

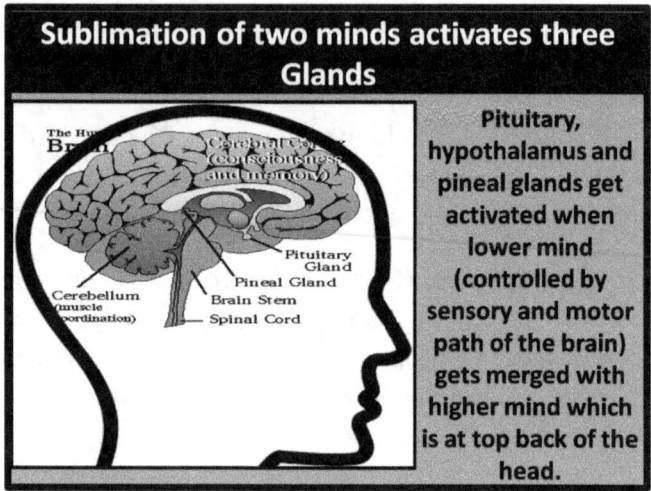

The image describes that when merger of lower and higher mind happens, the same will result the purification and activation of three glands (pituitary, hypothalamus and pineal glands). These glands play a vital role in psychic tunnel to explore the beneficial aspects for stability of lower mind at higher centers. These glands also help to accelerate the merger process of lower mind with higher mind.

Pituitary, hypothalamus and pineal glands get activated when lower mind (controlled by sensory and motor path of the brain) gets merged with higher mind which is at top back of the head. This means that middle brain where hypothalamus, motor and sensory path are available, plays a vital role in psychic tunnel for merger of two minds and make it (Bindu after union of higher and lower mind) stable platform (visualized as full moon).

The position of different glands in the human brain has been shown in the image which are inter connected and inter dependent for the better function of body and mind. The features and beneficial aspects of these glands have been described.

8.5.1 Pineal Gland

The main function of pineal gland is to make Nero-hormones which affect both levels of our existence that is brain and body. This clearly indicates that unless pineal gland is purified and the same becomes active, the Nero hormones will not be secreted. The same will not be effective at two existence of an individual that is body (where lower mind works) and brain (where higher mind works). Kriya yoga helps to secrete these hormones.

Melatonin, the principal product of the mammalian pineal gland, acts as an internal representative of nighttime. The secretion of melatonin is increased under light-dark cycles, with an increase in the dark period and a decrease in the light period the pineal gland may be able to directly sense the light. Immuno cytochemically, it is reasonable to believe that the pineal gland can be photo-receptive. The pineal was simply called 'folded retina', a variety of genes that are only expressed in eyes are expressed in the pineal gland as well.

The Pineal Gland is about the size of a pea, weighing little more than 0.1 gram and is in the center of the brain. It is the point of connection between the intellect and the body. It is located directly behind the eyes. At the age of seven or eight the pineal gland begins to degenerate in every child and the pituitary is unleashed. Because of this there is no balance because the pineal was not maintained in a healthy state when it began to degenerate. It is also known for "seat of the soul". The pineal gland is a photosensitive organ and an important timekeeper for the human body. In humans it affects sleeps patterns and is implicated in seasonal affective disorder.

The pineal gland is occasionally associated with the sixth charka. Extra doses of bright light can cause the pineal gland to produce less melatonin thereby eliminating some of the symptoms of SAD. This gland is activated by Light, and it controls the various biorhythms of the body. . In periods of darkness the pineal gland produces melatonin, a hormone that shows significant sedative properties.

The pineal gland has always been important in initiating supernatural powers. The pineal gland and the pituitary body must vibrate in unison, which is achieved through meditation and/or relaxation. The pineal gland situated at the top of the spinal column in the medulla oblongata. It is also known as the "Third Eye".

The image describes the important aspects of pineal gland. It provides many beneficial aspects in day to day life such as making us to have more learning capability and better memory storage. The image briefly sums up the beneficial aspects of pineal gland in materialistic life as well as in spiritual domain.

It speeds up our memory and learning abilities. In addition, it Enhances intuition, wisdom and creativity by utilizing the highest power of mind. The pineal gland is the seat of great power and potential for dynamic and vibrant life. This clarifies that pineal gland is very important gland (which normally gets dried up in common mass) in materialistic world. By activating the same we achieve best possible personality while dealing with people, object, place and situation.

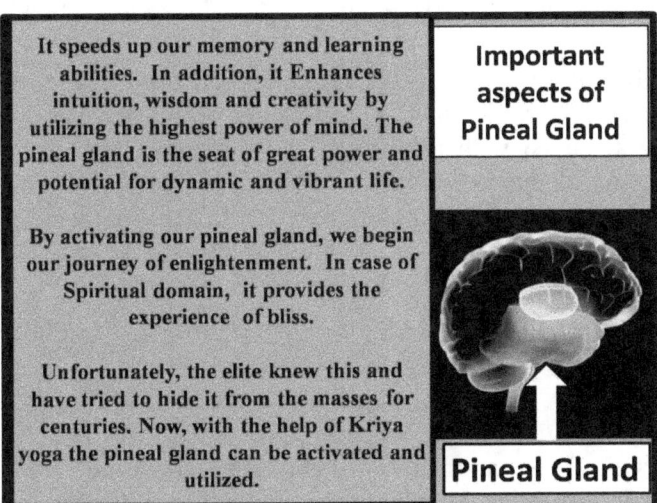

It speeds up our memory and learning abilities. In addition, it Enhances intuition, wisdom and creativity by utilizing the highest power of mind. The pineal gland is the seat of great power and potential for dynamic and vibrant life.

Important aspects of Pineal Gland

By activating our pineal gland, we begin our journey of enlightenment. In case of Spiritual domain, it provides the experience of bliss.

Unfortunately, the elite knew this and have tried to hide it from the masses for centuries. Now, with the help of Kriya yoga the pineal gland can be activated and utilized.

Pineal Gland

By activating our pineal gland, we begin our journey of enlightenment. In case of Spiritual domain, it provides the experience of bliss. This is an added feature of pineal gland to achieve the purpose of taking birth. Unfortunately, the elite knew this and have tried to hide it from the masses for centuries. Now, with the help of Kriya yoga the pineal gland can be activated and utilized.

8.5.1.1 Pineal gland crown (Turiya as centre of consciousness)

Beginning with the withdrawal of the senses and the

physical consciousness, the consciousness is centered in the region of the pineal gland. This happens when we develop our absolute consciousness (Brahm Chaitanya) as per Vedanta. At this juncture, the perceptive faculty and the point of realization are centralized in the area between the middle of the forehead and the pineal gland.

The trick is to visualize, very intently, the subtle body escaping through the trap door of the brain. This can also be achieved with the help of Jyoti Trataka (gazing of candle flame intentionally at inner part of the brain). Deep meditation is the best solution to achieve this kind of visualization.

8.5.2 Hypothalamus

There is a pathway from the retinas to the hypothalamus called the retino hypothalamic tract. It brings information about light and dark cycles to a region of the hypothalamus called the Supra Chiasmatic Nucleus (SCN). From the SCN, nerve impulses travel via the pineal nerve (sympathetic nervous system) to the pineal gland. These impulses inhibit the production of melatonin. When these impulses stop (at night, when light no longer stimulates the hypothalamus), pineal inhibition ceases and melatonin is released. The pineal gland is therefore a photosensitive organ and an important timekeeper for the human body.

The image describes the important features of hypothalamus. It is situated in front of brain stem and its complex network. The brain stem also contains a complex network of brain cells and fibers which runs through its entire length. The brain cells and fibers receive all the sensations here, and messages pass to the rest of the brain and works like alarm system. Hypothalamus is the important conveyer of the information in the brain.

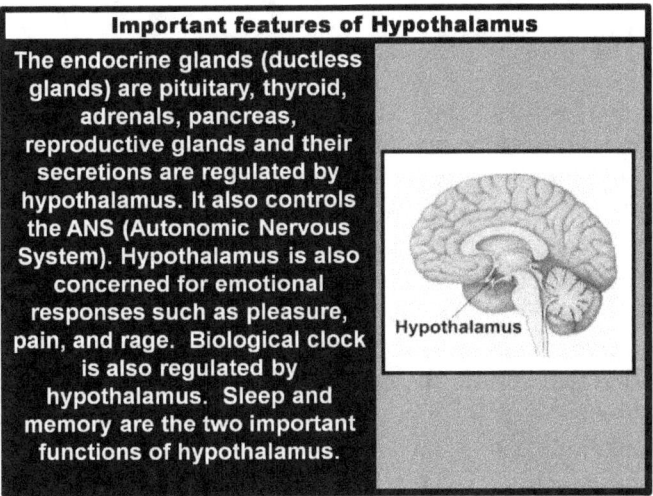

Important features of Hypothalamus

The endocrine glands (ductless glands) are pituitary, thyroid, adrenals, pancreas, reproductive glands and their secretions are regulated by hypothalamus. It also controls the ANS (Autonomic Nervous System). Hypothalamus is also concerned for emotional responses such as pleasure, pain, and rage. Biological clock is also regulated by hypothalamus. Sleep and memory are the two important functions of hypothalamus.

Hypothalamus

The image describes different kinds of endocrine glands. These glands are ductless and they are pituitary, thyroid, adrenals, pancreas, reproductive glands and their secretions are regulated by hypothalamus. It (hypothalamus) works as controller of these glands. The secretion of chemicals from these glands is regulated depending on the alarming situation (the demand of secretion to face the situation).

It also controls the ANS (Autonomic Nervous System). In turn, ANS regulate parasympathetic and sympathetic nervous system. This means hypothalamus is indirectly is the controller of PSNS and SNS. Hypothalamus is also concerned for emotional responses such as pleasure, pain, and rage. Biological clock is also regulated by hypothalamus. Sleep and memory are the two important functions of hypothalamus.

8.5.3 Relationship between pituitary and pineal gland

To activate the 'third eye' and perceive higher dimensions, the pineal gland and the pituitary body must vibrate in unison, which is achieved through meditation and or relaxation. When a correct relationship is established between personality operating through the pituitary body and the soul operating through the pineal gland, a magnetic field is created. The negative and positive forces interact and become strong enough to create the 'light in the head.' With this 'light in the head' activated, astral projectors can withdraw themselves from the body, carrying the light with them. The magnetic field is created around the pineal gland, by focusing the mind on the midway point between the pineal gland and the pituitary body. The creative imagination visualizes something, and the thought energy of the mind gives life and direction to this form.

The image describes the importance of pituitary glands for the development of mankind. This gland is also known as the Gland of Command (Agna chakra). Agna chakra commands five systems (circulatory, respiratory, digestive, excretory and central nervous system) of the body to regulate the physical and mental health.

For proper development of socio economy, environment, cultural, educational and spiritual aspects; we need adequate development of pituitary and pineal glands. This is because, pineal glands works as on- off switch for pituitary gland. Normally, common mass will not have the proper growth of pineal gland in the youth hood as it gets dried up. In that situation, pituitary will not get the proper impacts of pineal which is required for uplifting the lower mind at higher centers and also for merging the same with higher mind. That is why, the balance of these two minds is essential.

Importance of pituitary glands for the development of mankind

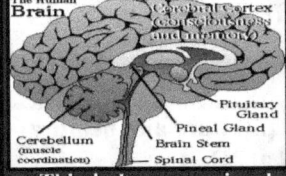

For proper development of socio economy, environment, cultural, educational and spiritual aspects; we need adequate development of pituitary and pineal glands. This is because, pineal glands works as on- off switch for pituitary gland. Normally, common mass will not have the proper growth of pineal gland in the youth hood as it gets dried up. In that situation, pituitary will not get the proper impacts of pineal which is required for uplifting the lower mind at higher centers and also for merging the same with higher mind. That is why, the balance of these two minds is essential.

Otherwise, inadequacy of pituitary and pineal glands, there would be growth of criminals and unrest society. Imbalance of inferiority complex among the youth and management people will not have the self control though; they will be having self esteem. It is important to note that pituitary gland alone guides the lower mind responsible for the physical need with the help of karma Indriya and Gyan Indriya. Whereas, pineal gland alone can guide the higher mind for thinking, planning, organizing, leading and controlling the mental work.

Both together will uplift the lower mental work of pituitary gland and higher mental work of pineal gland with proper justification to achieve overall development in the society.

8.5.4 Pituitary gland

The pineal gland works with pituitary through hypothalamus to control endocrine system of the body. This means pineal gland helps to activate pituitary, thyroid, pancreas, adrenal and reproductive gland. These glands are responsible for healthy physical and mental life.

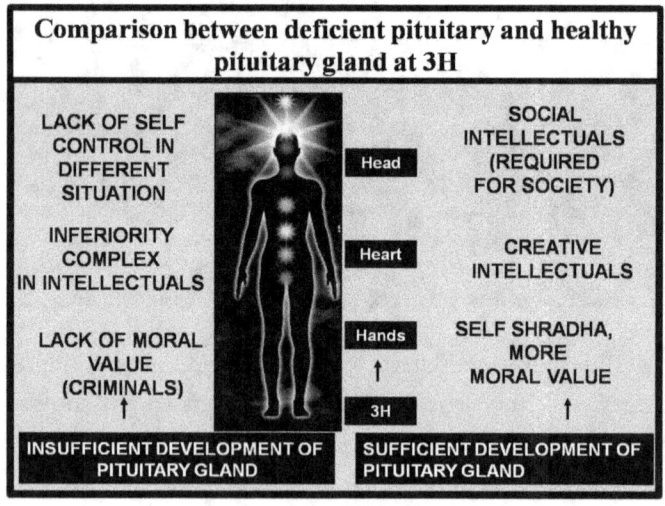

Pineal also controls the emotional state of the mind in head region (mental state) and dream & deep sleep in physical state. For understanding we can take pituitary gland as on switch and Pineal gland as off switch. Pineal gland produces a chemical in the brain that enhances meditative state. Neuro chemical and anthropological are the evidence.

In case of insufficient development of pituitary gland, there will be development of criminal attitude because of lack of moral value at Hands level. At Heart level, there will be inferiority complex among the intellectuals. Similarly, there will be lack of self control in different situations among the learned people.

The situation will be different if pituitary gland is properly functioning with the help of pineal gland. For example, at Hands level there will be inner development of better moral value and faith (Shraddha). Likewise, at Heart level the intellectuals will be more creative and also at Head level, the intellectuals will be working more for the society (social oriented); which is the need of the hour.

8.6 Meditation acquires the Theta state

Theta state of the brain wave helps to dive inside the unconscious mind where suppressed imprints along with Sanchit karma (collected imprints during evolution) exist. Normally, frequency of brain wave at theta state is about five CPS or below. This is achieved in meditation (Kriya yoga first and then meditation is continued).

At certain brainwave frequencies, a sense of ego boundary vanishes. In the theta state, we are resting deeply and still conscious. As the brain enters deeper states, our consciousness is less concerned with the physical state, our 'third eye' is active, and separation becomes natural.

To develop the 'Third eye', imagination, and visualization are important ingredients. To separate from the physical form, third eye development is helpful. Intuition is also achieved through third eye development. Knowledge and memory of astral plane are not registered in full waking consciousness, until the intuition becomes strong enough. Flashes of intuition come with increasing consistency when third eye is activated to a greater degree. Universal knowledge can also be acquired through intuition.

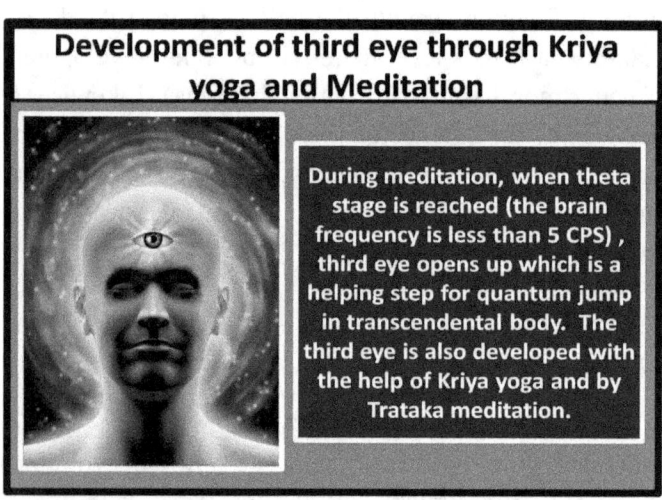

Development of third eye through Kriya yoga and Meditation

During meditation, when theta stage is reached (the brain frequency is less than 5 CPS), third eye opens up which is a helping step for quantum jump in transcendental body. The third eye is also developed with the help of Kriya yoga and by Trataka meditation.

The image describes the different methods of activating the third eye in brief. It also explains that theta state works as stepping stone for quantum jump while meditation. During meditation, when theta stage is reached (the brain frequency is less than 5 CPS), third eye opens up which is a helping step for quantum jump in transcendental body. The third eye is also developed with the help of Kriya yoga and by Trataka meditation.

9. CONCLUSION

Kriya Yoga is kept secret by many Yogic Institutions since beginning because it is very powerful and can be misused by the Sadhakas to harm the society. For example, Siddhi achieved in perfection of Kriya Yoga can be used or misused among the people of Society depending on remaining trace of six temperaments of Sadhaka.

Secondly, if not followed properly, the same (Kriya Yoga) may harm the individual in place of being as boon for spiritual development. The best boon of Kriya Yoga is to become "Divine", which can be a platform for Quantum jump in Spiritual domain (Transcendental domain).

This is perhaps, the probable stepping stones for the scientists of late19th and beginning of 20th century to discover (experience and witness) the function of Nature (Prakriti) to arrive Quantum theory. It is interesting to note that the nature (Prakriti) is the manager of Absolute

Reality (Permatma) for the creation of Universe with the help of mystic domain.

The function of nature (Prakriti) while creation of human system comes as a nucleus (Bindu) consisting five basic elements like Ether (Akash), Air (Vayu), Fire (Agni), Water (Jala) and Earth (Prithivi) from mystic domain in combination with inner instruments (Mana or Mind, Mana Buddhi or Intellect, Ahamkara or Ego and Chitta or Resultant space) and soul (regulator and controller of energy and space). During manifestation this Bindu (Nuclei) gets divided and known as higher & lower mind. The lower mind functions like anchor point for energy and space wherever it exists. Mostly the same (lower mind) exists at lower centers of the body.

Now the question arises whether two Bindu (Nuclei) can be sublimated? The answer is yes (positive). To have the clarity, better to know the different names of the two Bindu (Nuclei) given in Veda, Upanishad and Yogic scriptures. The first Bindu which is mostly called as a white Bindu is also known as Consciousness, Purusha, and Shiva (CPS). Likewise, the second Bindu which is known as red Bindu or rajas is also known as Energy, Prakriti, and Shakti (EPS). The possibility for the merger of the two Bindu namely Shiva and Shakti is examined and the same is described by the image in brief.

9.1 Whether lower and higher mental energy could be merged?

There are many methods to sublimate Shiva (higher mind or white Bindu) and Shakti (lower mind or red

Bindu) in Astang yoga. The sublimation is also possible through Karma yoga, Bhakti yoga and Gyan yoga. Among all the methods discovered so far, Kriya yoga seems to be an important one. In Kriya yoga, Maha mudra and Yoni mudra (or Shanmukhi mudra) techniques are suggested for sublimation of these two Bindu. The image describes the process in brief.

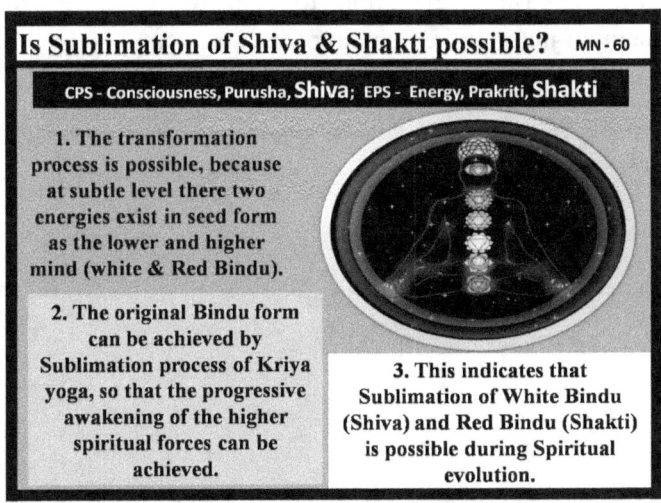

Is Sublimation of Shiva & Shakti possible? MN - 60

CPS - Consciousness, Purusha, Shiva; EPS - Energy, Prakriti, Shakti

1. The transformation process is possible, because at subtle level there two energies exist in seed form as the lower and higher mind (white & Red Bindu).

2. The original Bindu form can be achieved by Sublimation process of Kriya yoga, so that the progressive awakening of the higher spiritual forces can be achieved.

3. This indicates that Sublimation of White Bindu (Shiva) and Red Bindu (Shakti) is possible during Spiritual evolution.

The image describes that the transformation process is possible, because at subtle level there two energies exist in seed form as the lower and higher mind (white & Red Bindu). This means that the Shiva (higher mind) and Shakti (lower mind) are in the seed form and they can be merged if a technique is available to uplift the Shakti. It (Shakti) can be uplifted with the help of raising Apana prana and merging the same with prana. After merging, the same can be forced (with the help of flow of air) to reach up to white Bindu and then get merged.

The original Bindu form (at top back of the head) can be achieved by Sublimation process of Kriya yoga, so that the progressive awakening of the higher spiritual forces can be achieved. The steps described in Kriya yoga like Maha mudra and Yoni mudra is very useful for the sublimation. This indicates that Sublimation of White Bindu (Shiva) and Red Bindu (Shakti) is possible during Spiritual evolution to find the platform for quantum jump in the domain of transcendental body.

Brief about Prof. A.N. Pandey (Author)

Shri A.N.Pandey worked with Bhabha Atomic Research Center (DAE) as Senior Scientific Officer till 2006. He acquired wide experience & expertise in the field of project management.

To achieve the best possible performances, to have better inter-personal relation, to obtain total quality management and to achieve self-motivation forced Shri Pandey to go in quest of spirituality. He was equally interested in acquiring the knowledge & experience of "Ancient Indian Wisdom (AIW)" through reputed institutions of India in the field of Spirituality. He worked & developed a spiritual (Vedantic) model in association with SVYASA (Swami Vivekananda Yoga Anushandhana Sansthana), World Class Yoga University, Bangalore. He was also associated with Bihar School of Yoga, Simplified Kundalini Yoga (SKY), Vipassana Meditation, YSS (Yogada Satsang Society) and Brahma Kumari.

Presently he is heading a research institute known as "Spiritual Awareness Program (SAP)" at Hyderabad and responsible for developing many packages such as "personality development for student", "personality development for professional" and "professional development for manager". He has also developed packages for stress management, anger management, resistivity management, leadership, self motivation, time & mind management and communication skills in the background of spirituality (Yoga & Vedanta).

He visualized many simple and effective techniques such as science of breathing, development of subtle inner personality, relaxation in action and meditation in action by taking the themes of spirituality. SAP is engaged in solving other International problems related to sustainable development in the fields of crime, modern education, global economy, poverty, therapy, judiciary and political unrest.

Shri Pandey is visualizing a common platform for scientist and spiritual masters where they (scientist and spiritual masters) can come together to take each other findings (related to special theme of science and spirituality) to define the consciousness (supreme reality). This platform is important for both (scientist and spiritual master) are working to reveal the truth of creation in easy way.

He is author of many Books in the field of Killer Diseases, Management, Spirituality, Health Management and Social Reform. He has brought out many deeper Yogic concepts (from Veda and Upanishad) and made them easy to understand by the common mass. His books are available at Swami Vivekananda Yoga Prakashna (SVYP), Bangalore, India and also on Amazon.com (www.yogicconcepts.in). ∎